Building Healthy Communities
through Medical-Religious Partnerships

Building Healthy Communities

through Medical-Religious Partnerships

Third Edition

W. Daniel Hale, PhD
Richard G. Bennett, MD
Panagis Galiatsatos, MD
Johns Hopkins University School of Medicine

JOHNS HOPKINS UNIVERSITY PRESS   BALTIMORE

This book was brought to publication through the generous assistance of the William S. Perper Foundation.

Johns Hopkins University Press
2715 North Charles Street
Baltimore, Maryland 21218-4363
www.press.jhu.edu

Library of Congress Cataloging-in-Publication Data

Names: Hale, W. Daniel (William Daniel), 1950– author. | Bennett, Richard G. (Richard Gordon), 1956– author. | Galiatsatos, Panagis, 1987– author.
Title: Building healthy communities through medical-religious partnerships /
    W. Daniel Hale, Richard G. Bennett, Panagis Galiatsatos.
Description: Third edition. | Baltimore, Maryland : Johns Hopkins University Press,
    2018. | Includes bibliographical references and index.
Identifiers: LCCN 2017044507 | ISBN 9781421425801 (pbk. : alk. paper) | ISBN
    1421425807 (pbk. : alk. paper) | ISBN 9781421425818 (electronic) | ISBN
    1421425815 (electronic)
Subjects: | MESH: Community Health Services—organization & administration |
    Health Education | Religion and Medicine | Community-Institutional Relations |
    Patient Advocacy
Classification: LCC RA564.8 | NLM WA 546.1 | DDC 362.1/0425—dc23
    LC record available at https://lccn.loc.gov/2017044507

A catalog record for this book is available from the British Library.

Special discounts are available for bulk purchases of this book. For more information, please contact Special Sales at 410-516-6936 or specialsales@press.jhu.edu.

Johns Hopkins University Press uses environmentally friendly book materials, including recycled text paper that is composed of at least 30 percent post-consumer waste, whenever possible.

Contents

Foreword

I was delighted when Dan Hale asked me to provide the foreword to this, the third edition of *Building Healthy Communities through Medical-Religious Partnerships*. As a physician and a theologian, I have had a career that has encompassed what—on the surface—seems to be two divergent fields: medicine and theology. Hence, I understood the important work that this book would describe. I was not disappointed.

This book is one of the most practical health-related books for those affiliated with religious communities that I have ever read. The authors intend this book to be easily read by nonmedical persons, and they have succeeded in producing a work that is both highly informative and user-friendly. Information about various physical and mental conditions, especially what they are, how they are treated, and what happens when they are not prevented or treated in a timely fashion, is valuable for all of us, and the authors present this material in a highly accessible manner. With each condition is information on what local congregations can do and examples of congregations that have actually done so, providing the reader with encouragement that his or her congregation could do likewise. As a bonus, each of these chapters includes up-to-date websites for more information.

Yet, this book is not merely another listing of the conditions and diseases that impact us in the twenty-first-century United States. There is also information about how to speak with a health professional so that the encounter is of optimal benefit to all concerned; managing medications so that they can be used to their greatest effectiveness; supporting family **caregivers** so that they can both care for themselves and for their loved ones; and community and national resources that congregations can access.

I believe this book to be a valuable resource for every congregational leader and member interested in the intersection of faith and health. The information provided can be used by *any* congregation—regardless of its location, polity, or socioeconomic mix—because there are always members with the various conditions described in the book, even (and especially) if these conditions are not discussed openly (e.g., mental health issues). In *each* congregation—again, regardless of location, polity, or socioeconomic mix—there are also members who need to have conversations with health professionals, are taking medications, are serving as caregivers to family members, or need access to accurate medical information. This book is invaluable for these purposes as well. That is why the practical suggestions offered for what congregations can do give this book its authenticity. The authors have been party to that which they describe.

As a physician, I find that the medical information in this book resonates with me. In my experience, people often perish before their time because of lack of accurate information about potential and existing health threats, or their lack of trust in medical institutions to "do right" by them. As a native Baltimorean who grew up in proximity to many of the houses of worship described in this book, I have witnessed that many congregations trust their clergy and lay leaders far more than they trust health care professionals (no matter how kind and caring the latter are), another reason to include religious leaders (ordained and lay) as partners in community health. Health is not just a private matter; the health of an entire community depends on the health of each of the citizens. Unfortunately, this is a lesson that is taking much too long for us all to learn.

And, as a pastoral theologian who now has the responsibility for teaching and training those already in ministry and those who aspire to some form of ministry, I have heard not only the discouraging stories of health care inequities in my students' neighborhoods but also the soaring success stories of congregations making a difference—oftentimes, starting with one person and then extending beyond the walls of the physical structure that houses the congregation. These accounts of success are certainly more than "feel good" stories; they are the essence of religious faith because—as *all* world religions teach—we are to do to others what we would have others do to us. May this belief become more than a catchphrase; may it become the reality by which we all live.

Patricia Fosarelli, MD, DMin
Associate Dean, St. Mary's Ecumenical Institute
Assistant Professor, Johns Hopkins University School of Medicine

Preface

The first edition of *Building Healthy Communities through Medical-Religious Partnerships* documented our work in the 1990s, when we became convinced that partnerships between health care systems and religious congregations had tremendous potential to meet many of the difficult challenges associated with an aging society in the United States and with the concomitant growth in the number of people with chronic conditions at the time. Over these years, we had witnessed enthusiastic clergy and congregational volunteers, supported by dedicated medical professionals, offering programs that helped people maintain their health, independence, and dignity, which we described in the original edition. The second edition presented some updating of this work, and over the past decade we have expanded our initiatives to include more age groups. Currently, we have become even more convinced of the valuable role that medical-religious partnerships can play in addressing the health care needs of communities throughout the country.

Although most of our original work occurred in Florida, we have been especially impressed over the last six years with partnerships in Baltimore, Maryland, and the surrounding region that show how these programs can address the serious **health disparities** that continue to impact so many of our communities. Our work in Baltimore has also demonstrated that these partnerships can serve a valuable role in the training of physicians and other health professionals, including pastoral care providers, by giving them opportunities to move beyond the walls of the hospital and, thereby, gain a better understanding of the importance of the effects of **social determinants of health**.

> We have been especially impressed how these programs can address the serious health disparities that continue to impact so many of our communities.

Because of a generous bequest from the William S. Perper Foundation in 2012, funding has been available to us to support an annual symposium focused on our work. These events have allowed us to share our excitement about many of the new initiatives developed in Baltimore in past years, and

also inspired us to develop new ones. We have been pleased that our enthusiasm for this work has been reciprocated by the many clergy and their
congregants, as well as health and human services professionals who have
come together each year to participate in the Perper Symposia. These symposia have alternated between Baltimore and New York, focus on faith-based
connections, and offer examples of effective programming along with information on helpful resources. The William S. Perper Foundation, strongly
committed to building medical-religious partnerships, also has provided
funding to help support the publication of this book and other materials
that can be used in congregational health programs.

For readers who are new to our work, we hope you already share our belief
that health care systems, medical professionals, and religious congregations
can and should join forces to minister to the health needs of their community. We hope that the third edition of this book provides not only strong
support for this belief but also detailed information and advice on programs
that have proven successful in a diverse group of congregations and communities over the past 25 years. We report on innovative medical-religious
partnership programs organized by various health systems, some with ties to
religious organizations (e.g., Catholic and Seventh-Day Adventist), but others
with no current or historical connection to any national or local religious
group. And we share stories of health programs offered by congregations
representing a wide range of faiths and denominations—African Methodist
Episcopal, Baptist, Catholic, Episcopal, Greek Orthodox, Jewish, Lutheran,
Methodist, Muslim, Presbyterian, Seventh-Day Adventist, and Unitarian
Universalist—and from various parts of the country.

The book opens with an introduction that provides an overview of some
of the most serious health challenges our country faces and why partnerships between health care systems and religious congregations are able to
address these challenges. Clergy and lay leaders interested in seeing how
a congregational health program can complement existing ministries and
programs will find outstanding examples in the first three chapters of part
1. In chapter 1, we report on a congregational health program that has been
going strong for almost 25 years. This is followed by two chapters illustrating
how medical-religious partnerships can address health disparities affecting
the two largest minority groups in the United States—African Americans
and Hispanics/Latinos. The programs in these three chapters also illustrate

how an effective and vibrant congregational health ministry can be run at virtually no expense to the church.

Health care professionals and religious leaders who have questions—and perhaps even doubts—about the amount of interest in congregational health programs and the types of programs they believe are needed will find answers to many of these questions in the survey results in chapter 4. Elsewhere in that chapter we present a brief summary of the basic principles and methods of preventive medicine and illustrate how they can be incorporated into congregational programs. Chapter 5 provides an overview of the strategies that congregations can employ to link people with valuable health information and resources through proactive health education programs.

Part 2 focuses on specific medical topics across the entire age span—from infant care to end-of-life care. Assisted by a panel of distinguished experts from the Johns Hopkins Medical Institutions, we provide, in a concise format designed specifically for individuals with little or no background in health care, the latest information about the most common conditions that lead to preventable death and disability and the treatments for each. These chapters also include suggestions for congregational programs and examples of such programs, and at the end of each chapter, we provide information on additional resources.

Part 2 also contains strategies and resources that individuals can use to reduce their own health care risks and effectively manage their medical conditions with the goal of maintaining functional independence. Topics covered include communicating with health care providers, lifestyle modifications, medication management, home safety, and **advance directives**. The final chapter in this part introduces Called to Care, an initiative at Johns Hopkins that recognizes the need to support family caregivers—health care's "invisible workforce." One of the major aspects of Called to Care is the work with religious congregations, providing them with the expertise and resources they need to assist family caregivers and their loved ones. Several of the chapters in the section include brief guides that can be reproduced and shared with interested persons. These guides are also available in PDF format on the book's companion website (www.hopkinsmedicine.org/jhbmc/building-hcp) and can be downloaded and copied.

Part 3 includes chapters reporting on two innovative programs that have been developed since the publication of our second edition, each related in a meaningful way to our earlier work forging connections between medical institutions and faith communities. Chapter 22 introduces a Community Partners Clinical Pastoral Education program that has medical-religious partnerships as a key component, providing trainees with a better understanding of how their work as spiritual care providers can go well beyond the walls of a hospital. Chapter 23 reports on a medical residency program at Johns Hopkins that offers interns and residents an opportunity to participate in a health education program for volunteers from religious congregations. Enthusiasm for this program among these physicians contributed to the creation of Medicine for the Greater Good, a medical education initiative targeting health disparities locally and globally that was cofounded by Dr. Panagis Galiatsatos, one of this book's authors.

Finally, part 4 provides information on resources that can be used by any individual or organization interested in developing medical-religious partnerships. Chapter 24 offers guidance on how to identify and access local agencies or organizations, while chapter 25 offers descriptions and contact information for national organizations that offer valuable health education materials. The book concludes with a glossary (terms that appear in boldface in the text may be found in the glossary) and a reference list.

The programs and materials presented in this book are by no means exhaustive. Religious congregations can sponsor many other programs, and religious and medical institutions can work together in a multitude of ways to enhance community health. To facilitate the sharing of new models and programs, we will use this edition's companion website to highlight and catalog successful medical-religious partnership programs as they come to our attention. Additionally, PowerPoint slides and other materials that can be used in congregational health programs are available on the website, and we will use the site to highlight important developments in medicine and health care that could be of interest to those working to improve the health and wellness outcomes among the congregants and patients of neighboring faith-based and health care institutions.

Given the ongoing challenge in our country to improve health outcomes for individuals, as well as address known population health challenges and disparities, we remain more convinced than ever that there has never been a better time to explore innovative and collaborative efforts to minister to the health needs of communities. We are in the midst of a fundamental change in the way people are conceptualizing and organizing health care. Health care leaders are increasingly aware that they need to reach out to the community through trusted institutions, and religious leaders are learning they can ask for assistance and support from medical institutions. We encourage you to take the initiative to bring medical and religious communities closer together.

Acknowledgments

We could not have written a book about community health partnerships without the assistance and goodwill of many people. First and foremost, we want to express our appreciation for the steadfast support and encouragement of the late Mr. and Mrs. William E. O'Neill. The programs we initially designed 25 years ago could easily have gone no further than the idea stage if it were not for their generosity and efforts on our behalf. Firmly convinced of the value of programs in which medical institutions and professionals work in partnership with faith communities, they established a charitable foundation that continues to provide support for these programs. We are also indebted to their daughters, Mary O'Neill Clement and Paula O'Neill Bower, the other members of the O'Neill family, especially Tim and Cindy O'Neill, and the individuals who have served as officers of the O'Neill Foundation for Community Health—Barbara Pearson, Bette Heins, PhD, Bill Allen, JD, MDiv, and Lisa Ford Williams—for their continued support.

We also want to acknowledge and express our gratitude to the trustees of the William S. Perper Foundation—James Coleman, James Purdy, and Kevin Sunkel—who have provided generous support that has enabled us to expand our work to Maryland, New York, Washington, DC, Pennsylvania, and Delaware.

A number of health care leaders who have worked directly with us in key roles as we developed and implemented our programs deserve recognition for their contributions. These include Bill Griffin and Jeff Feasel (Halifax Health), Daryl Tol (Florida Hospital), Leana Wen, MD, and Heang Tan (Baltimore City Health Department), Reverend Debra Hickman, MDiv (Sisters Together and Reaching), and Reverend Gregory Johnson (EmblemHealth).

We would especially like to thank the Johns Hopkins faculty and staff who contributed to this edition by helping us update, revise, and improve the clinical chapters:

John R. Burton, MD
Professor of Medicine
Johns Hopkins University School of
    Medicine

Margaret S. Chisolm, MD
Associate Professor & Vice Chair for
    Education of Psychiatry & Behavioral
    Sciences
Member, Miller-Coulson Academy of
    Clinical Excellence
Johns Hopkins University School of
    Medicine

Deidra C. Crews, MD, ScM, FASN, FACP
Associate Professor of Medicine,
    Division of Nephrology
Johns Hopkins University School of
    Medicine

Tom Finucane, MD
Professor of Geriatrics
Johns Hopkins University School of
    Medicine

Sherita Hill Golden, MD, MHS
Hugh P. McCormick Family Professor of
    Endocrinology and Metabolism
Executive Vice-Chair, Department of
    Medicine
Johns Hopkins University School of
    Medicine

Torie Grant, MD
Research and Clinical Fellow of
    Pediatrics Allergy and Immunology
Johns Hopkins University School of
    Medicine

Nadia N. Hansel, MD, MPH
Associate Professor of Pulmonary and
    Critical Care Medicine
Associate Dean of Research, Johns
    Hopkins University School of
    Medicine
Chair, Johns Hopkins Bayview Scientific
    Advisory Board
Johns Hopkins University School of
    Medicine

Kai Hartman-Shea, MSW, LCSW-C
Director of Social Work
Johns Hopkins Bayview Medical Center

Christopher Marano, MD
Assistant Professor of Psychiatry and
    Behavioral Sciences
Johns Hopkins University School of
    Medicine

Jane Marks, RN, MS
Division of Geriatric Medicine and
    Gerontology
Johns Hopkins University School of
    Medicine

Tessa K. Novick, MD, MSW
Research and Clinical Fellow of
    Nephrology
Johns Hopkins University School of
    Medicine

Sarah Polk, MD, ScM, MHS
Assistant Professor of Pediatrics
Co-Director, Centro SOL
Johns Hopkins University of School of
    Medicine

Katherine Shaw, MD
Instructor, Departments of Internal
  Medicine & Pediatrics
Assistant Program Director
Internal Medicine-Pediatrics Urban
  Health Residency Program
Johns Hopkins University School of
  Medicine

Eugene Shenderov, MD, PhD
Research and Clinical Fellow of
  Oncology and Hematology
Johns Hopkins University School of
  Medicine

David Shih Wu, MD
Assistant Professor, Division of General
  Internal Medicine
Johns Hopkins University School of
  Medicine
Director, Palliative Care
Johns Hopkins Bayview Medical Center

Sammy Zakaria, MD, MPH
Assistant Professor of Medicine
Associate Program Director, Johns
  Hopkins Bayview Internal Medicine
  Residency
Assistant Director, Johns Hopkins
  Bayview Cardiac Intensive Care Unit
Johns Hopkins University of School of
  Medicine

The expertise they brought to this work has made for a better book, for which we are most appreciative. Finally, we thank Kimberly Monson for her many contributions as program coordinator for the Healthy Community Partnership, and Robin Coleman, our editor, for his encouragement and guidance.

Building Healthy Communities
through Medical-Religious Partnerships

Introduction

For most of the past 100 years, hospitals have been places where people in the United States were treated for acute illnesses related to infections and the need for surgery. With improvement in public health and operative techniques over the past 50 years, now the majority of hospitalizations for adults are related to acute **exacerbations** (worsening) of underlying chronic diseases.[1] At present, almost one-half of American adults have at least one chronic disease, and seven of the top ten causes of death are chronic diseases. Two of these chronic diseases—heart disease and cancer—account for almost half of all deaths. Particularly alarming is the recent finding that for the first time in 20 years, the life expectancy of Americans has actually declined.[2]

What makes chronic diseases so challenging is that much of the care for people with chronic diseases is provided not in hospitals or physicians' offices but in the homes of the affected individuals. And most of that care is provided not by physicians and nurses but by the individuals themselves. Medical professionals continue to play essential roles with respect to chronic diseases, particularly for acute exacerbations, but the responsibility for the day-to-day management of most of these diseases—monitoring the conditions, using medications correctly, implementing and then sustaining recommended lifestyle modifications—rests largely with the affected individuals themselves or family members who assist them at home in their care. Thus, health care organizations committed to improving the health of their communities must find ways to reach out to those who have chronic diseases and others who are at risk for chronic diseases and to

For the first time in 20 years, the life expectancy of Americans has actually declined.

provide them with the information and support they need to manage their conditions and to use medical services in a timely and appropriate manner.

Another serious challenge facing health care systems is the increasing racial and ethnic diversity of our communities. It is expected that by 2020, minority ethnic and racial groups will make up 40 percent of the US population, and by 2030 that number will climb to almost 45 percent.[3] At the same time that we are becoming more diverse, the health status of most people who belong to a racial or ethnic minority group continues to lag behind that of the rest of the population. For example, non-Hispanic/Latino black adults are at least 50 percent more likely than non-Hispanic white adults to die of heart disease or **stroke** prematurely (before the age of 75), and the **prevalence** of diabetes is 70 percent higher among Hispanic/Latino adults than among non-Hispanic white adults.[4] Increasingly, health care systems will have to develop programs that are responsive to the special medical needs of various minority groups and that reflect an understanding of the values and traditions of these groups. Clinicians working with members of minority groups will need to pay special attention to the issue of trust because mistrust of medical institutions and professionals can be a significant barrier to the delivery of needed services.

So how can health care organizations, most of which are experiencing severe financial pressures, address these challenges? Where can they find the resources to educate large numbers of people about chronic diseases? How can they reach people in the community who have no ties to the health care system and are not even aware that they may have a chronic condition? How can they tailor programs to meet the needs of increasingly diverse communities? And how can they overcome the mistrust of medical institutions that exists among some groups?

There is a way for health care organizations, large and small, to address these challenges. But they cannot do it by themselves. To reach and maintain contact with people, providing them with the information and resources they need to make good decisions about their health and medical care, health care organizations need partners. They need to work closely with institutions that are deeply rooted in the community and are trusted by people in the community. Health care organizations need to develop alliances with institutions that have a strong tradition of caring for others and that attract people who identify with this tradition.

Religious congregations–churches, synagogues, mosques, and temples—

clearly fit this description. They have the community resources and communication networks that hospitals need. Just as important, they have the altruistic traditions and values that are at the heart of community-based health programs. No community institutions are better suited to serve as partners for hospitals. This is especially true for addressing the health needs of older adults and families who have the responsibility of caring for older adults. Whereas most children and adolescents can be reached through school-based health promotion programs and most young and middle-aged adults can be reached through work-site initiatives, religious institutions are the one place where large numbers of older adults regularly gather.

Over the past 25 years, we have witnessed the tremendous impact that medical-religious partnerships can have on the health of communities, reaching large numbers of people who had not been reached by other health programs. We have seen enthusiastic members of religious congregations work closely with health care organizations and medical professionals to organize programs focusing on the management of specific diseases, such as high blood pressure and diabetes. Through such programs, participants have been alerted to the need to identify these conditions as early as possible to minimize future complications. Some programs have helped people recognize and respond promptly to the earliest signs of a heart attack or stroke, and other programs have instructed people how to use advance directives to maintain control over their medical care if they become incapacitated because of injury or illness.

Valuable information about **hospice** care has been presented by health professionals and reinforced by clergy. Reminders about screenings and vaccinations and information about where these services are available have been printed in congregational bulletins and announced during worship services and other congregational gatherings. Through programs like these—programs that have brought together the expertise and resources of the medical community with the dedication and energy of volunteers from religious congregations—people have become more knowledgeable about important medical issues and the medical services available in their communities as well as more skillful in working with their own physicians and other health care providers.

We have been particularly impressed with the effectiveness of medical-religious partnerships in reaching minority communities. When health care organizations have demonstrated a sincere interest in working with members of predominantly minority congregations to address their concerns in a culturally sensitive fashion, this interest has been met with enthusiastic support from clergy and lay leaders. They have welcomed representatives of health care organizations to their communities and offered valuable advice about how to break down barriers that have kept many from receiving health services.

One of the encouraging aspects of programs built around medical-religious partnerships, and one of the reasons they have great potential to address some of the most serious health care challenges of the twenty-first century, is how much can be accomplished without straining the financial resources of health care organizations. Most hospitals and medical centers already have the materials, services, and personnel needed to offer programs to religious congregations. They do not need to create new departments or hire additional personnel.

Believing as strongly as we do in the need for communities throughout the country to forge medical-religious partnerships, we have prepared a book that can be used to introduce the basic idea of these partnerships to medical and religious leaders—to help them "catch the vision" and to serve as a manual or guide for health programs. In writing this book, we have drawn not only on our experience but also on that of hospital administrators, physicians, nurses, pharmacists, chaplains, clergy, and congregational volunteers who have been involved in medical-religious partnerships in many communities.

Health care systems can begin building partnerships with congregations in several ways. Most hospitals already have a broad network of contacts with the religious leaders in their own communities, and these local clergy regularly serve on ethics committees or provide pastoral care for persons who have been hospitalized. Many larger hospitals employ full- or part-time religious professionals as chaplains who become active members of the health care team and typically provide oversight and management for the hospital's volunteer clergy staff. These individuals can be engaged to begin an outreach program designed to strengthen the ties between the hospital and multiple faith communities in the neighborhoods served by the hospital. Inaugural programs can be structured as evening seminars that provide an overview of the contents of this book and review the resources that the hospital can make available to interested congregations. Alternatively, a wider net can be cast, and copies of the book can be sent to local congregations with a letter inviting interested recipients to call for more information.

Special attention and efforts may be needed when hospitals seek to establish relationships with congregations in parts of the community where members may be doubtful or even suspicious about the motives behind a hospital's new outreach program. In these situations, it is advisable to make direct contact with a telephone call and an offer to visit clergy and lay leaders at their own local house of worship to describe this opportunity more fully and to begin building a trusting relationship that can serve as the foundation for programs that will empower all members of the community to better care for themselves, their families, and their neighbors.

I THE RELIGIOUS CONGREGATION AND HEALTH CARE

1

Healing Body, Mind, and Soul

A Model for Health Ministry

The Reverend Dr. Jeffrey Sumner had approached the summer of 1999 full of optimism and enthusiasm as he worked with members of the congregation to prepare for Vacation Bible School and various other summer programs. He had no reason to think that he might have a serious medical condition. As far as he could tell, he was in excellent health, and everything seemed to be going well at church and at home. Although his first few years at Westminster By-The-Sea Presbyterian Church in Daytona Beach, Florida, had been stressful as he helped the congregation heal the deep wounds and divisions that had occurred prior to his arrival, the last few years had been especially gratifying. The congregation had doubled in size during his tenure and now offered ministries and programs that drew people of all ages. Sunday morning worship services were well attended, Sunday school classrooms were full, and so many young families had joined the church that the nursery had been expanded to three rooms. It wasn't just on Sundays that people came to the church. Almost every day the buildings were buzzing with activity.

He had no reason to think that he might have a serious medical condition.

Life was good at home, too. There were no unusual or particularly difficult stresses. In fact, his wife, Mary Ann, and their three children all seemed to be thriving. He could look at his family and his work with a great deal of satisfaction. Life was, indeed, good.

Feeling as well as he did physically and emotionally, Dr. Sumner could easily have gone several more years without discovering he had a serious medical problem had he not stopped by the church fellowship hall on that morning in June to participate in a health **screening**. This screening, open to the wider community as well as to members of the congregation, was offered as part of Body, Mind, and Soul, the health ministry developed in collaboration with a local hospital and led by volunteers from his congregation. Fortunately, he did attend the screening, though his primary motivation was simply to show support for the program. And even then he almost escaped testing. His busy schedule had kept him from being present at the beginning of the screenings, so by the time he arrived, all of the risk assessment forms had been used. He graciously offered to forgo the testing, because he was certain he did not have any health problems, but the nurse coordinating the program insisted that she go to her car to get a form for him. She felt that it was important for him, as a congregational leader, to go through the testing.

After giving him time to complete the risk assessment form, the nurse drew a small sample of his blood to be tested. But a few minutes later, instead of giving him the results, she told him that she needed to run the test again because the equipment might have malfunctioned. After the second test was completed, she reported back to him that she had encountered the same problem and wanted her supervisor to run a third test. Only after this third test was Dr. Sumner given the results, and they were not what he had expected. The nurse discreetly informed him that she was concerned about what she had found. Each of the three tests had shown a blood sugar level of over 350, well above what was considered normal. His cholesterol level also was abnormally high. While not conclusive, these results led her to suspect that he had diabetes. She then briefly explained what it meant to have diabetes and why it was important that he begin treatment as soon as possible if he had it. She strongly recommended that he see his family physician to have tests run that could yield a more certain diagnosis.

Dr. Sumner was in shock as he left the fellowship hall, numb from the news that he might have diabetes. How could this be? How could he feel so good and yet have a condition that could wreak havoc throughout his body? Wanting to know for sure if he had diabetes, he called his family physician later that day. Dr. Jennings agreed that diabetes seemed likely and ordered blood tests for the following morning that would be more conclusive. When the results came back, there was no more doubt about the diagnosis. Dr. Sumner had **type 2 diabetes** and would need to begin treatment immediately.

The treatment plan that Dr. Jennings outlined at Dr. Sumner's next appointment was different from what many patients expect from their physicians and what would have been recommended had Dr. Sumner been diagnosed with an infection or another acute illness. He was given a prescription for a medication that would help him control the diabetes, but Dr. Jennings made it clear that the medication would be only one part of the overall treatment regimen. There was no quick and easy fix for diabetes. It was a chronic condition that would always be a part of Dr. Sumner's life, and it would require his daily attention. His blood sugar would need to be checked three times a day, and he would be the person in charge of that monitoring. An effective treatment regimen also would include significant changes in diet and daily routines, and here again he would bear the responsibility for implementing and maintaining these changes.

Dr. Jennings supplemented his explanation of diabetes and his treatment recommendations with printed materials that explained in more detail just how important diet and exercise would be in controlling diabetes, but he knew that even these handouts would not provide all of the information Dr. Sumner would need or answer all of the questions that were sure to arise. For this reason, he strongly recommended that Dr. Sumner enroll in a course on diabetes offered by the hospital.

Heeding his doctor's advice, Dr. Sumner contacted the hospital, where he learned that he would be expected to bring Mary Ann with him to all of the classes. Although she did not have diabetes, it would be important for her to learn about the disease and what she could do to help him monitor and control it. Mary Ann, who already had purchased several books on diabetes for the family, readily agreed to join him.

One of the first things they learned from the course instructor was just how harmful diabetes could be if not brought under control. They learned about the many serious long-term complications that could develop, including blindness, heart disease, stroke, kidney failure, amputations, and nerve damage. Dr. Sumner was especially concerned about the risk of amputations and loss of vision. He could not imagine what it would be like to continue in his vocation if he were unable to read or to move about easily.

Although the instructor wanted to impress on those attending the course the serious risks associated with diabetes, her purpose was not to scare them. Rather, it was to empower them by giving them the knowledge and skills they would need to gain control of their diabetes. She explained how the failure of their bodies to produce or appropriately use **insulin** resulted in abnormally high levels of **glucose** in the bloodstream that over time would do serious damage to parts of their bodies. To avoid these damaging effects, they would need to monitor their blood glucose levels regularly and adopt eating habits and exercise routines that could keep their blood glucose levels in a safe range. She showed them how to check their blood sugar and then had them practice doing it. For those who needed insulin to control their diabetes, she explained how and when to take it. They learned what to eat, how much to eat, and when to eat. With her guidance, they discovered how to prepare meals that would be healthy as well as tasty. She also stressed the importance of regular physical activity and of establishing an exercise routine that fit their schedules and interests.

There was a lot to learn, but by the end of the course Dr. Sumner's anxiety about diabetes was largely gone, replaced by a sense of confidence that he would be able to bring his diabetes under control. There was no question that his life was going to be different in many respects now that he had a chronic disease, but he emerged from the course convinced that his life would still be a full, active one as long as he took good care of himself.

Next came the real challenge for Dr. Sumner—translating his newly acquired knowledge about diabetes into a course of action. Because consistently following treatment recommendations involves changing habits and routines that are firmly established and often highly pleasurable, this can be a difficult hurdle for individuals with diabetes. What can make this even more challenging is that family members, coworkers, and friends may not understand and support their efforts. Fortunately, this was not the case for Dr. Sumner—at least not at home. After the initial shock of hearing that their father had diabetes, his children decided to educate themselves about his illness and do what they could to help him maintain his health. For example, as soon as they understood the importance of diet in controlling diabetes, they willingly joined with their father in preparing and eating healthier meals. And when they learned that their father had decided to begin a regular exercise routine of long walks in the neighborhood, they bought him a portable tape player (later upgraded to an iPod) so that he could listen to his favorite music along the way.

Dr. Sumner found that support and encouragement came from his church family as well. Thanks in large measure to the many health seminars and discussions held at the church, there was a spirit of openness and trust about medical issues among members of the congregation. They had become more comfortable discussing health concerns that previously they might have shared only with family members. Dr. Sumner had encouraged this openness, recognizing that speaking openly about a feared issue usually relieved much of the anxiety and frequently led to helpful suggestions and offers of help from others. Now it was his turn to share his medical concerns with members of the congregation and to ask for their understanding as he made certain changes in his life. He did this by writing the congregation a letter that he read to them before a Sunday worship service and subsequently printed in the church's monthly newsletter.

Members of the congregation, now aware of the medical challenges their minister faced, responded with kind words and deeds. Several who had diabetes shared their stories with him and offered encouragement. A teenage girl from church who had diabetes visited him to demonstrate how she measured her blood sugar and to talk about how she coped with diabetes. Her fearless and confident approach bolstered Dr. Sumner's confidence. The parishioners in charge of congregational meals began checking with him to make sure that at church dinners there were food choices that would allow him to stay on his diet. Members who invited Dr. Sumner into their homes for a meal did the same. Many members unobtrusively checked in with him from time to time to be sure he was taking good care of himself.

By the end of the summer, Dr. Sumner, who as a Presbyterian minister was used to passionately sharing the gospel of Jesus Christ, found what he called his "second gospel": that through proper monitoring, awareness, and partnerships with health providers, people in congregations and communities can live longer and healthier lives when armed with knowledge and opportunities for healthy life choices.

As Dr. Sumner reflected on the experiences in the months following his diagnosis, he realized just how important the church's Body, Mind, and Soul program had been to him and to so many others. Through the information and resources the program had brought into the congregation, he and the members of the church had learned valuable lessons that could help them prevent serious injuries and illnesses, detect diseases while they were at a treatable stage, manage chronic conditions, and find relief from many of the burdens of caregiving. Several of these lessons were clearly illustrated in his recent experiences.

Looking and feeling healthy does not necessarily mean that you are healthy.
   Just because he was free of pain and full of energy did not mean that he was free of disease. It had been easy for him to lull himself into a

false sense of security about his health simply because he was feeling good.

Easy access to health screenings and **preventive medicine** *can increase the use of these services.* His busy schedule often got in the way of proper preventive care, as it does with many people. It had been much easier to stop by the church for a screening than it would have been to get to the lab at the hospital or an outpatient clinic.

Successful treatment for most chronic conditions requires patients to become well informed and actively engaged in their medical care. He had learned that he would bear the responsibility for the day-to-day monitoring and management of his diabetes, and to do so, he needed to become knowledgeable about the disease and its treatment.

Good medical care is built around a partnership between patients and their health care providers that allows for the free flow of information in both directions. To provide an accurate diagnosis and effective treatment plan, his physician needed him to share all aspects of his life that might contribute to his condition or serve as barriers to effective treatment; and for the treatment to be successful, his physician needed to explain the diagnosis and treatment strategy in clear, understandable terms.

Coping with a chronic illness is easier when you are open with family and friends. The support, cooperation, and encouragement he had received from his family and the congregation made it easier to follow his doctor's treatment recommendations and to cope with the emotional dimension of diabetes.

Body, Mind, and Soul

The health screening at which Dr. Sumner learned he had diabetes was just one part of Body, Mind, and Soul, the comprehensive health ministry at Westminster By-The-Sea Presbyterian Church. This popular ministry had grown out of an innovative community health education program sponsored by a nearby hospital. Hospital administrators and physicians at Halifax Health Medical Center had long recognized the need in their community for more education about disease prevention and illness management. Every day they saw people coming through their doors with serious medical problems that could have been averted if they had taken the right steps or at least sought treatment before the disease had reached an advanced stage. They saw others who had been properly diagnosed and received appropriate treatment initially but then failed, for one reason or another, to follow through with the treatment recommendations they had received. The hospital administrators and medical professionals knew they needed to find a way to reach out into the community with the information and resources that would enable people to maintain their health and to use the hospital and other medical services in a timely and appropriate way. They needed a systematic approach that provided stronger ties, more continuity, and greater support.

When hospital administrators and several key physicians learned of a successful community health education program in Baltimore that involved a medical center's reaching out into the community through religious congregations, they decided to develop a similar program in Daytona Beach and the surrounding communities. Their program, like the one in Baltimore, would rely largely on volunteers from congregations willing to be trained as "lay health educators." With guidance from physicians at the Johns Hopkins University School of Medicine, they created a curriculum focused primarily on common chronic conditions—**hypertension**, heart disease, cancer, diabetes, **depression**, and **dementia**. Course material included information on the prevalence of each of these conditions, the reasons they often went undetected, the risk of complications if these conditions went untreated, and the steps people could take to prevent or at least gain control over these conditions. They also covered medication management, influenza and pneumococcal **vaccinations**, prevention of accidents and falls, and advance directives. Once the curriculum was established, they had no trouble finding physicians, nurses, pharmacists, and other health professionals affiliated with the hospital willing to serve as instructors and then provide ongoing support for volunteers as they developed their congregational programs.

With the curriculum and instructors in place, the next step was to recruit volunteers from local congregations. This was done by contacting clergy and inviting them to join with the hospital in developing congregational programs. Those who were interested were asked to identify one or two members of their congregation who would be interested in being trained as lay health educators. It was explained that the program would give volunteers the information and tools they needed to coordinate health education seminars, screenings, and support groups in their congregations. They also would learn about the various medical services and be equipped to serve as liaisons between their congregation and the hospital.

Twenty-five volunteers participated the first time this course was offered, meeting at the hospital two hours each week for eight weeks. When the course was completed, there was enough interest among local congregations for the course to be offered twice more. By the end of the first year, 59 volunteers from religious congregations and retirement communities had completed training as lay health educators.

Nancy Force, the volunteer from Westminster By-The-Sea Presbyterian Church, was like most of her classmates in the lay health educator program in that she had no formal training or experience in health care. What she did have was good organizational skills, an eagerness to reach out to people in need, and experience caring for her late husband during the chemotherapy and surgeries he endured as he battled cancer. By the time she had completed the course, she was ready and eager to start organizing health programs in her congregation. Working closely with Dr. Sumner and members of her congregation and sometimes with members of nearby congregations, she developed a series of programs covering what she had learned during her training. The enthusiastic response of the congregation and community to these programs was truly gratifying. Programs were well attended, often drawing a third or more of the audience from outside the congregation.

Unlike some programs that are popular when first offered but then fade away over time or come to an end when the original leader leaves, Body, Mind, and Soul grew in popularity and had become such an integral part of the overall ministry of the church that when Nancy Force needed to step down as coordinator, there was no question that the program would continue. Tina Buck, an elder in the church who was employed at that time by a large health care organization, continued the program and added new topics. Later, Helen Chandler, a nurse and elder in the congregation, took over and served as coordinator for several years. And when she left this position to head up another church program, Alexis Fortune stepped in and kept the program running strong.

Shortly after Body, Mind, and Soul celebrated its twelfth anniversary, Dr. Sumner sat down with me (WDH) to review the program's offerings and to discuss the many ways he felt the program had benefited members of the congregation and others from outside the church who had attended some of the offerings. He started by going over some of the topics that had been covered, summarizing the key points that had been emphasized by speakers and in the materials that often were handed out at seminars or included in congregational bulletins and newsletters.

Heart Disease. Dr. Sumner easily recalled a number of important points covered in the programs and materials devoted to heart disease. One was that heart disease remains the number one cause of death for women as well as for men, something that surprises many people. The importance of recognizing the earliest signs of a heart attack and then taking prompt action was stressed. Handouts listing warning signs of a heart attack were distributed and discussed, with attention being called to the fact that not all individuals experience crushing chest pain. As for prompt action, **cardiopulmonary resuscitation (CPR)** instruction was arranged for one session, and people were advised to call 911 immediately rather than trying to drive themselves or a loved one to the hospital and also to chew an aspirin while awaiting the paramedics' arrival. Programs and materials also emphasized that changes in lifestyle—particularly a low-fat diet, regular physical exercise, and stopping smoking—along with careful monitoring and control of cholesterol and blood pressure, could greatly reduce their risk of a heart attack.

> **Heart disease remains the number one cause of death for women as well as for men.**

Stroke. As with heart disease, programs and materials placed an emphasis on early detection and quick action. People were encouraged to think of strokes as "brain attacks" requiring immediate care. Lists of warning signs were distributed and reviewed, and the role of high blood pressure as a major risk factor was stressed. Special note was made of the fact that people could have dangerously high blood pressure and not be aware of it—thus, the importance of having it checked regularly. Lifestyle factors that could increase the risk of stroke also were reviewed.

Cancer. When we came to the topic of cancer, Dr. Sumner reported that the emphasis on early detection, something underscored in almost all programs and materials on the topic, had a special meaning for the congregation. Within a period of less than 18 months, two young men in the congregation, both in their thirties, had died of **melanoma**. Still feeling these tragic losses, members of the congregation were eager to learn about the methods for early detection of cancer, including **colonoscopies**, **mammograms**, and breast self-examinations. In seminars and the accompanying material, common misconceptions about these methods were directly addressed and corrected. And with respect to the prevention and early detection of skin cancer, the congregation not only spread the word among members but joined in sponsoring an annual community-wide event that raised awareness of the importance of screenings and also raised funds for a foundation that supported research on melanoma.

Diabetes. One of the major points emphasized in programs and materials was that in as many as one-third of adults with diabetes, the condition goes undetected and untreated. Coupled with this startling statistic was information about how untreated diabetes puts individuals at risk for a number of conditions that can cripple or kill, including heart disease and stroke. Symptoms that otherwise might be ignored, such as thirst, blurry vision, and fatigue, were listed, and the importance of maintaining a healthy diet and weight was emphasized.

Depression. One of the major goals of the programs on depression was to reduce the stigma that is still too often associated with mental illness. Dr. Sumner reinforced this message every chance he had, encouraging people to think of depression much as they think of other medical conditions and not as a sign of personal weakness. Another key point emphasized was that in most cases depression could be successfully treated through medication and/or psychotherapy, and that they should discuss their symptoms and concerns with their health care provider. Suggestions for recognizing symptoms and how to reach out to people who might be experiencing depression also were given.

Dementia. Much of the information on dementia addressed the issue of the tremendous burden **Alzheimer's disease** and other forms of dementia can place on family caregivers, who may feel that it is their responsibility to provide all of the care for a loved one or who may be unaware of community agencies that offer various forms of assistance, including respite care. Caregivers were urged to avail themselves of resources the church and other organizations offered. Also discussed was the value of having dementia diagnosed in its earliest stage because that allows patients to participate in the planning for their care during the later stages.

Palliative Care and Hospice. The programs on **palliative care** featured information on the services of local hospice organizations, with special attention given to common misconceptions about hospice care (e.g., that it is only for people with cancer or AIDS, that it is only for the final days or weeks of life) that often interfere with the timely and appropriate use of these services. Another issue addressed was the importance of advance directives that allow individuals to maintain control of their care even if an injury or illness should prevent them from communicating their wishes. In addition to providing information about advance directives, the church keeps in the office a supply of the Five Wishes form developed by Aging with Dignity and gives members the option of having a copy of their completed form kept at the church.

Managing Medications. Advice and strategies for effective management of medications were offered at programs led by pharmacists and also as part of programs focusing on specific illnesses (e.g., heart disease, depression). A key point emphasized in all programs was that every health care provider a person sees should be aware of every medication that individual is taking, including over-the-counter medications. It also was emphasized that people should not discontinue a prescribed medication without first discussing the matter with their health care provider.

Home Safety. One of the key messages of programs on preventing falls and accidents was that individuals should not be reluctant to use assistive devices (e.g., canes, walkers, and wheelchairs) if they have a condition that increases their risk of falling. This message was reinforced by Dr. Sumner with individual members whenever he thought it might be appropriate and by the church's program of loaning walkers and wheelchairs to members. He even told those with walkers to think of them as their "everlasting arms" and to "lean on them" even when they felt self-conscious about using them. Other programs and materials on accident prevention and securing homes from intruders and scam artists provided advice and simple ways to make people's lives safer.

On-Site Screenings. One of the principal points emphasized in several of the educational seminars was that it was possible for people to be unaware that they have a potentially serious medical condition. Therefore, it is important for them to be screened for various conditions, even if they are experiencing no symptoms. To reinforce this point and to remove some of the obstacles that often get in the way of people scheduling screenings at their doctor's office or a hospital laboratory, Dr. Sumner and the leaders of Body, Mind, and Soul decided to arrange for screenings to be conducted at the church and, whenever possible, in conjunction with regularly scheduled services and programs. An excellent example of making a screening easily available is the church's program of screening for skin cancer. Participation in the screenings, conducted annually and offered immediately after the Sunday morning worship service by local dermatologists, is always high (50 to 90 individuals), and several members have discovered that they had a suspicious lesion that warranted further medical attention. Body, Mind, and Soul also arranges for blood pressure screenings and hearing tests to be conducted. These, like the skin cancer screenings, are offered immediately after the Sunday worship service during the church's fellowship hour, when members and visitors mingle and enjoy light snacks. Body, Mind, and Soul also sponsors screenings for diabetes, like the one where Dr. Sumner first learned he had diabetes, and cardiac risk factors (e.g., cholesterol and triglycerides). These are done in collaboration with the hospital's laboratory and typically offered on weekdays rather than Sundays.

On-Site Preventive Care. With approximately half of the congregation in the age group most at risk for serious complications from influenza (65 years of age or older), the leaders of Body, Mind, and Soul decided they wanted to do more to educate members about the importance of vaccinations. Working with the county health department, they have arranged to offer vaccinations at the church every fall. Each year this is preceded by an educational campaign to inform members of the benefits of influenza vaccinations and to correct misconceptions about its dangers. A similar program for vaccination against pneumonia is offered at the church every other year.

Congregational Care Teams. This program, established following a presentation by a local hospice organization, brings together small groups of volunteers to provide nonmedical care and support for individuals whose ability to live independently is threatened by their frailty or medical condition. A team's activities often include transportation, shopping, and light housework, with each team dividing up the workload so that no member is overwhelmed by caregiving responsibilities. Complementary congregational programs have used speakers from the Council on Aging to describe sources for financial and physical assistance.

Support Groups. The church is home to Alcoholics Anonymous, Al-Anon, and Gamblers Anonymous support groups. Dr. Sumner noted that the church does more than provide space for these support groups. In each case, there is at least one member of the congregation who, because of the openness and trust that exists among church members, has been willing to speak publicly about his or her struggles with an addiction and to encourage others who are battling an addiction to seek help and support.

Exercise and Weight-Reduction Groups. Body, Mind, and Soul has hosted several programs demonstrating proper exercises for back pain and cardiovascular strengthening. In addition, the church has offered a weekly "Meditation and Stretching" class to help people with their physical, emotional, and spiritual challenges. One of the serendipitous developments Dr. Sumner has witnessed is members, convinced of the health benefits of regular physical activity, finding others in the congregation who enjoy the same type of activity and want to have a partner or group to join with them. Similar pairings or groups have formed among members interested in weight reduction.

As we neared the conclusion of our conversation, Dr. Sumner emphasized just how much this program means to the congregation. It is not simply the number of people attending seminars or participating in screenings that impresses him. It is also the conversations he hears among members as they gather for Sunday school classes or visit with each other during the fellowship hour. It is not unusual for them to be discussing their latest blood pressure readings or cholesterol levels or their plans for a colonoscopy or mammogram, and doing so with an informed understanding of these topics. Their church has come to be known not only as a reliable source of Christian teaching but also as a reliable source of health information.

   The program's influence is also evidenced throughout the week in homes and doctors' offices and hospitals throughout the Daytona Beach area. People who have participated in the offerings of Body, Mind, and Soul carry with them a well-placed sense of confidence about health matters. Medical professionals and the health care system are no longer as intimidating as they had been. These participants believe in the value of regular medical visits, and they know how to make the best use of the time with their health care providers. They have a greater appreciation of the need to understand and follow the treatment recommendations of their providers. They know what symptoms or physical sensations signal a call to 911 or a trip to the hospital's emergency department. Participants have a belief in their ability to reduce their risk of premature illness, disability, and death, and they act on this belief. They are eager to share what they have learned through these programs with family, friends, and colleagues. There is no doubt in Dr. Sumner's mind and in the minds of dozens of health professionals who have participated in the church's health ministry that this program, built around

Congregations can be inviting, encouraging, and informing, empowering people to take proactive steps in the care of their bodies, minds, and souls.

partnerships with health care organizations, continues to have a significant and far-reaching impact on the congregation and community.

As we prepared this third edition of *Building Healthy Communities through Medical-Religious Partnerships*, I was eager to question Dr. Sumner again. Was Body, Mind, and Soul still an important part of Westminster By-The-Sea Presbyterian Church's ministry to its members and the community? Had it been possible for the church to sustain this health ministry for more than two decades? I was very gratified to learn that Body, Mind, and Soul was, indeed, still going strong. Members of the congregation and individuals from the community at large continue to count on the program for reliable health information and screenings. Dr. Sumner remains a strong supporter of congregational health ministries, believing that through such programs "congregations can be inviting, encouraging, and informing to parishioners and to the general public, empowering people to take proactive steps in the care of their bodies, minds, and souls. Medical-religious partnerships can build important bridges and relationships that are a boon to communities."

2

Transforming Lives
and Communities

Members and visitors who attend worship services at Southern Baptist Church in Baltimore, Maryland, can count on hearing a powerful message delivered by the church's dynamic pastor, the Reverend Dr. Donté Hickman. But on some Sundays, they may hear an additional message—one given by a health professional who has been invited by Dr. Hickman to speak to this largely African American congregation about a medical topic that he strongly believes is important for them to understand and, in many cases, to act on. A good example is the Sunday that Dr. Thomas Cudjoe, a Johns Hopkins physician, spoke on hypertension (high blood pressure), a serious medical condition that affects more than 50 percent of African Americans. Dr. Cudjoe explained how high blood pressure, if undetected and untreated, can have devastating—even deadly—consequences. To illustrate this, he shared with the congregation a personal story about a recent trip to his hometown in Georgia. His visit was not for a family reunion, retirement celebration, or wedding, but for the funeral of a favorite aunt who had been a major influence in his life. This beloved woman, who had been a pillar in the community, had died from a stroke caused by her high blood pressure. But Dr. Cudjoe went on to explain that high blood pressure doesn't have to lead to a stroke, heart attack, or kidney disease—that there is good news for those who have learned they have high blood pressure. This is a condition that can be managed and controlled. To illustrate the hopeful part of his message, Dr. Cudjoe shared the story of another aunt who had been diagnosed with hypertension more than 20 years

> Hypertension (high blood pressure) is a serious medical condition that affects more than 50 percent of African Americans.

before. Her response to this diagnosis has been to carefully monitor it, always taking advantage of the automated blood pressure monitors in pharmacies and grocery stores, and taking the prescribed medication religiously. Dr. Cudjoe concluded his message by urging everyone to do exactly what his aunt is doing—check their blood pressure regularly and, if they find that they do have high blood pressure, work with their health care provider to control it. Additionally, because this is such an important health issue for so many, especially in the African American community, he asked them to share what they had learned with family and friends.

The people who heard Dr. Cudjoe speak that Sunday didn't have to wait until their next medical appointment to act on his advice. They didn't even have to wait until Monday. Because of a partnership Dr. Hickman and the church had developed with Johns Hopkins Medicine, all they had to do was to stop by the fellowship hall where there were several volunteers ready to check blood pressures. And, if they discovered that their blood pressure was high, there were doctors and nurses available to offer advice and guidance. At the conclusion of the worship service, the congregation was reminded of this opportunity by Dr. Hickman, who strongly encouraged them take advantage of it, just as he was going to do.

The Sunday program on high blood pressure is just one of the many health programs Southern Baptist Church offers members of the congregation and residents of the adjoining neighborhood, and there is no question that these programs are greatly needed. The church is located in one of the poorest and most distressed neighborhoods in Baltimore. Ample evidence of the serious health needs of this community can be found in the Neighborhood Health Profiles produced by the Baltimore City Health Department. There is a separate health profile for each of the city's 55 Community Statistical Areas (CSAs), or clusters of neighborhoods. If you were to look through the profile for the CSA where Southern Baptist Church is located, you would see that the average life expectancy is only 66.9 years, ranking this neighborhood all the way at the bottom—55th out of the 55 CSAs. (In neighborhoods just a few miles away, the average life expectancy is 20 years greater.) You also would see that this neighborhood has a very high percentage of children in single-parent households (83 percent), a large number of families living in poverty (30 percent), limited green space (12 percent), large areas that are a food desert (48 percent), and high levels of violence (a homicide rate twice that of the city's and a nonfatal shooting rate three times that of the city's).

Dr. Hickman speaks eloquently and passionately about the importance of the church actively addressing the health, economic, and social ills of the community—being a powerful force for healing and justice. Dr. Hickman also talks about how the neighborhood is similar in many respects to what his own life was like years ago. There was a time when his life seemed to be in shambles and beyond repair. Given the path he was on then, one that included hardcore drugs and crime, the outlook for him was grim. There were no dreams of building a successful career or even escaping the confines of his impoverished neighborhood.

It would be easy to characterize Dr. Hickman's life at that time as a life without hope. He seemed destined for failure. But not everyone saw it that way. In addition to his mother, who never gave up on her son, there was the judge he faced after being arrested for his third offense. When this jurist looked at the young man in front of him, he saw someone who still had the potential to turn his life around, and who deserved one more chance. That act of faith prompted young Donté to reengage with the church, and when he did, he found preachers who also believed in him and encouraged him to dream about a better life, one that could take him well beyond the neighborhood where he was living and allow him to develop and utilize his gifts. So he began dreaming about a new life, and he started a journey that would take him far from Baltimore before he would eventually return to his hometown in 2002 to serve as pastor of Southern Baptist Church.

The neighborhoods around the church already were in decline by 2002. Everywhere you looked there were abandoned properties. The major employers had left the community, as had most retailers, and crime rates were among the highest in the city. The situation was so bad that a few years after he arrived, the local newspaper wrote an article about this neighborhood and described it as "a neighborhood without hope." But Dr. Hickman didn't see it that way. Instead, he saw a neighborhood that still had potential. Just as the judge had refused to give up on him years before, he was unwilling to give up on this east Baltimore neighborhood. And he believed that Southern Baptist Church could serve as a beacon of hope and an agent of transformation for the neighborhood. It could play a critical role restoring lives as well as properties.

Addressing the physical and emotional needs of residents certainly would have to be a key part of the church's ministry in this community. Dr. Hickman knew that many residents had never been given the information and resources they needed to maintain their health. He was aware of people who had their legs amputated because they had never learned how to control diabetes. Others never even knew they had high blood pressure until they had a crippling stroke. There were those who had lost their sight because **glaucoma** had gone undetected and untreated. Each year there were individuals hospitalized for serious, life-threatening complications of the flu, complications that likely could have been prevented had they been vaccinated. He knew of men who had died of prostate cancer and women who had died of breast cancer at relatively young ages because their cancers had not been detected early enough to be treated effectively. Many who suffered from heart disease, the number one killer in the neighborhood, had never been taught what they could do to reduce the risk of developing this disease. Even if they did have an understanding of the importance of a proper diet and regular physical activity, it was difficult to travel to a grocery store where they could buy affordable healthy foods, and concerns about the safety of their neighborhoods prevented them from getting regular physical activity. And often, just as Dr. Hickman had done growing up, many residents of the neighborhood did not seek medical care until an illness or injury was so severe that they needed to go to the emergency room.

Dr. Hickman was particularly concerned about the older adults in the congregation and community. He felt that too many seniors had been forgotten. Their voices were not being heard, and they were not receiving the attention and respect they deserved. He also knew that many of them were living in isolation, unable to leave their homes because of physical limitations or concerns about their safety. Additionally, this is the age group most likely to be facing the challenges of multiple chronic conditions—arthritis, high blood pressure, heart disease, diabetes, and diseases of the eye, among others.

Because of his own experience growing up, Dr. Hickman also had special concerns about the young people in the congregation and community. As he talked with them, he heard repeatedly about the impact violence was having. Most of these young people had been surrounded by violence for most of their lives. Almost everyone had a family member or close friend who had been a victim of violence, and many of these young people themselves had been assaulted. At night, it was common to hear gunshots and wailing sirens. Something else he noticed as he met with children and teenagers was that many of them did not seem to have any constructive plans for the future. They didn't talk about college or careers. They didn't have dreams of a better life. Dr. Hickman understood that without a vision for the future, they had little incentive to take good care of themselves and to avoid risky situations and activities.

Dr. Hickman knew that it would take innovative ideas, significant resources, strategic partnerships, and strong leadership on his part to address these various health concerns. The church would need to find new ways to reach out into the community, and he and the church leadership would have to find creative ways to tie health initiatives to Sunday worship services and other regularly scheduled activities, much as was done with Dr. Cudjoe and the blood pressure screenings. For example, as flu season approached, the church worked with doctors and the Baltimore City Health Department to arrange for free flu vaccinations immediately after the Sunday worship service. Once these arrangements had been made, Dr. Panagis Galiatsatos, a Johns Hopkins physician, was asked to speak for a few minutes during the Sunday worship service to talk about the importance of being vaccinated against the flu and to correct some of the misconceptions that often keep people from getting vaccinated. He strongly encouraged the congregation to take advantage of the free vaccinations. Later in the service, Dr. Hickman took the time to reinforce Dr. Galiatsatos's message and to urge people to get vaccinated, saying that he would be doing so immediately after the service, and he wanted others to follow his lead.

Another example of bringing health information and resources to people coming to church for religious services involved the church's spring revival, "A New Wine Outpouring." On the opening night of the revival, a Johns Hopkins Medicine mobile health unit staffed by a physician and physician assistant was parked at the entrance to the church, and people coming to revival services were invited to have their blood pressure checked and to talk with the physician or physician assistant about any health concerns they had. Also, those who attended the revival services were encouraged to register for workshops that would be offered the following Saturday during what was being called the "New Wine Overflow." Among the most popular workshops offered were ones on nutrition and stress management.

One of the most significant ways Dr. Hickman and Southern Baptist Church have addressed the needs of older adults in the community has been to develop affordable housing for them. This came in the form of an apartment complex built across the street from the church. This complex not only gives seniors safe, secure residences but also provides them with common areas where they can socialize and exercise with fellow residents and attend classes on a variety of topics. One of the popular classes offered focuses on how to prepare healthy meals, something that can be challenging for older adults who have special dietary concerns. Additionally, the facility includes more than just apartments. It also houses the Mary Harvin Transformation Center. This center, leased and operated jointly by Johns Hopkins Bayview Medical Center and the Johns Hopkins Hospital, has offices and a classroom, where health programs and courses are offered to residents from the senior apartments and residents of all ages from the neighborhood. For example, ophthalmologists and staff from the Wilmer Eye Institute at Johns Hopkins have used this space to conduct glaucoma and vision screenings. Because of the interest this generated, an additional program on eye diseases—glaucoma, **cataracts**, and **macular degeneration**—was held. Other popular programs offered in this facility have included "ask a doc" sessions on medications, arthritis, diabetes, lung disease, foot care, depression, and social isolation. The Mary Harvin Transformation Center also is home to some of the programs and services offered by the Johns Hopkins Department of Spiritual Care and Chaplaincy. Reverend Christopher Brown, the department's community chaplain, has an office there, and the classroom is the site for their "Caring for the City" course that offers clergy from throughout Baltimore opportunities to learn more about how faith communities and medical institutions can work together to address spiritual, physical, and emotional needs.

The Mary Harvin Transformation Center also is used to address one of the most important social determinants of health—unemployment. Professionals from the Johns Hopkins Health System's human resources department regularly offer programs and services to those in need of employment. This includes regularly updating community members about the types of opportunities available at both Johns Hopkins University and the Johns Hopkins Health System, reviewing resumes and job histories, offering sessions on interviewing skills and resume writing, assisting with the application process, and conducting some screening interview sessions on-site.

To address the psychological impact of violence on members of the congregation and community, especially the youth, Dr. Hickman has worked with Dr. Anita Wells, a clinical psychologist and member of the congregation, and Reverend Brown to develop programs that provide individuals the opportunity to share their experiences, gain a better understanding of the various ways these experiences are impacting their lives, and develop effective coping strategies and strong social support networks. Another program for the youth is mentoring—making sure that children and teenagers have at least one adult who firmly believes in their potential and is willing to work with them to help realize that potential.

The best way to understand what these programs and the partnership between Southern Baptist Church and Johns Hopkins have meant to a community with so many needs is to read the words of Dr. Hickman.

On the first Sunday in January 1992 I was invited to preach at the Southern Baptist Church. I had never traveled that far into East Baltimore. Nevertheless, I found a very warm and spirit-filled church that received me wholeheartedly that Sunday morning. So much so, that the pastor, Reverend Nathaniel Higgs, announced after my sermon that I would become the next pastor of the Southern Baptist Church. I was just 21 at the time and headed to Wiley College in Marshall, Texas. But 10 years later it happened. Pastor Higgs called me in Philadelphia, where I was pastor in a church and asked if I would succeed him as pastor of Southern Baptist. I agreed, and he invited my wife and me to a McDonald's, where he said we could order whatever we wanted.

In that very moment was the irony of my journey in ministry. I was being invited to become the pastor of a "mega" church and was working out the details at a local fast food restaurant. It was further confirmation that God does some of his highest work in the humblest of places and people. Southern Baptist had no idea that they were not just calling a young man with a Bachelor's degree from Wiley College, a Master of Divinity degree from Garrett Evangelical Theological Seminary, and a Doctor of Ministry from Wesley Theological Seminary. But they were calling a young man who started with a GED because he had been expelled from three Baltimore City public high schools. They were calling a young man who had been arrested three times for auto theft. They were calling a young man who had consumed and distributed hardcore drugs. I was the product of an inner city community and a single-parent home. I had been physically abused by my stepfather, who placed me in a tub of scalding hot water at the age of 3 that almost killed me. Instead, I suffered unexplainable and humiliating burns to my feet and buttocks that trouble me even to this day. Yet, the psychological trauma, impoverished environment, and seemingly hopeless situation didn't kill the hope nor dim the light within me to pursue my higher calling to become a preacher.

I was able to hear God's call after having to go to court for my third offense and being found guilty of all charges. But the judge at that time looked at me and said that I didn't look like a hardcore criminal. He said that I looked like a young man who could go to college and make something out of his life. So he gave me one more chance. And I took it by first going back to church and beginning a relationship with Christ. And then I began to sense a different passion within myself—a passion to become a minister. And that passion drove me to cultivate and expose myself to people and places that could heal me from the brokenness of my past. I wanted to be healthy mentally, physically, and emotionally.

By the time I became pastor of Southern Baptist, I knew what my assignment was. It was clear to me, ministering in a community of dilapidation and disinvestment, that the vision was to restore people as we rebuilt properties. After gaining an understanding and appreciation of my own personal odyssey and transformation, the same possibilities resonated within me for the health and growth of the church and the community. How to do it became the question. I then developed task forces within the church to do a study of the community to determine the real and felt needs of the community. We then began to see some of the serious health disparities within the community—mental and behavioral health, HIV/AIDS, substance abuse, educational **Through this medical-religious partnership, we are able to build relationships of trust.** challenges, unemployment, and poor physical health. We then envisioned a community transformation center that would house community health services that would seek to address the holistic health needs of the community so that they could take advantage of job opportunities, affordable housing, mixed-use property development, and amenities that we would build and provide. For me, it was important that we not just address the physical structural dilapidation but the human capital within the community. And I have discovered that the same passion that drove me to become healthy and transformed is the same passion that drives me to see a community that was dubbed "a neighborhood without hope" get the help it needs to be healed and transformed. And I have been very fortunate to find a partner that has been nearby all along in Johns Hopkins Medicine and Johns Hopkins University.

This partnership ironically was conceived at my mother's 60th birthday party through a chance encounter with Dr. Dan Hale, special advisor to Dr. Richard Bennett, president of Johns Hopkins Bayview Medical Center. He engaged me about opportunities to develop a partnership with their Called to Care program.

This soon expanded to a discussion of additional ways we could partner. I had a vision, but little did I know that Dr. Hale and Johns Hopkins would be the provision of life to a community that has been on long-term life support. Through this medical-religious partnership, we are able to build relationships of trust between Johns Hopkins Medicine and the community. In so many instances, people in the inner city have been so distressed and oppressed that they don't trust institutions to help them to heal or prevent unnecessary illnesses. But they do trust their churches and their pastors to, as the psalmist says, "lead them beside the still waters and make them to lie down in green pastures." It's because of partnerships like this that we can facilitate healing beyond the altar of prayer. While I believe in miracles, the manifestation is through medicine, prevention, diagnosis, counseling, and nutrition. These are the areas where true transformation takes place. And I am glad that the two have become one for this community of East Baltimore, and a model for urban centers everywhere.

3

Embajadores de Salud

If you attend a Sunday Mass at Baltimore's Sacred Heart of Jesus Catholic Church—better known to members of the growing Latino community in the surrounding neighborhoods as Sagrado Corazón de Jesús—you are likely to be given, along with the church bulletin, a handout with information on high blood pressure or diabetes or another important medical topic. If you are there for one of the well-attended Masses offered for Spanish-speaking parishioners, you would find this health information is provided in Spanish. Then, if you were to stop by the parish hall while the young Latino children are in their religious education classes, you might discover the parents of these children engaged in a lively discussion about heart disease or common medication issues with a local physician fluent in Spanish. And if you drop by the church on a Saturday morning, you might be invited to join a group of young adults, teenagers, and children having fun as they exercise. These are only a small part of a larger, vibrant health ministry that developed when the church entered into a partnership with physicians and other health professionals from an academic medical center just a mile away.

This medical-religious partnership began in 2012, when Dr. Gerardo Lopez-Mena approached the church's priest, Father Robert Wojtek, and expressed interest in offering Spanish-language health education classes at the church. At the time, Dr. Lopez-Mena was a junior (second-year) resident in the internal medicine residency program at Johns Hopkins Bayview Medical Center. Many of the patients he saw in the hospital and outpatient clinics were recent immigrants from Mexico and several Central American countries who spoke little or no English and, because of the language barrier, had a limited understanding of their illnesses and the recommended treatments.

It wasn't unusual for him to see patients who had failed to recognize early warning signs of a disease and thus did not seek medical care until they were seriously ill, often suffering major complications that could have been avoided if they had sought treatment earlier. And he also found that, once ill, they had difficulty navigating the health care system.

Although Dr. Lopez-Mena's recent experience providing medical care to Spanish-speaking patients was an important factor in his decision to propose a church-based health education program, it wasn't the only factor. There also was a very personal element. Like many physicians, Dr. Lopez-Mena's decision to pursue a career in medicine can be traced back to his childhood years and the illnesses that brought him into frequent contact with doctors. Born prematurely, he spent his first few weeks in a neonatal intensive care unit. Then, for many years, there were the frequent visits to the clinic he and his mother had to make as they struggled to control his asthma. But the path that led from those early clinic visits to a successful career as a physician was quite different from the paths of most of his colleagues, and it included experiences that would give Dr. Lopez-Mena a special understanding of what life was like for many of his Latino patients.

Dr. Lopez-Mena grew up in a largely low-income, Latino community in southern California. The medical care he received was not provided in the private offices of a physician, but in the free clinic available to those who did not have health insurance or the financial resources to pay for their care. He vividly remembers the long lines of people waiting to see one of the clinic doctors and the fear in his mother's face when she thought they might not make it to the front of the line. He also remembers her happiness and the gratitude she felt when they were able to be seen by a doctor.

Dr. Lopez-Mena also confronted a number of significant challenges as he pursued the education he knew he would need if he were to achieve his dream of becoming a doctor. Living in a low-income neighborhood, he attended crowded public schools, where he and his fellow classmates had to rely on outdated textbooks. But crowded classrooms and inferior school materials were often the least of his concerns. More worrisome were the gangs, drugs, and violence he encountered almost every day as he walked to school. Fortunately, Gerardo had a loving and supportive family that helped shield him from many of the temptations and dangers of the neighborhood and that provided the guidance he needed to stay on the path he had chosen. His parents, both of whom had come from small Mexican villages and had only an elementary school education, were determined that their five children would go to college and have successful careers. They also instilled in their children a sense of service, empathy, and community, something that Gerardo would carry into his work as a physician and that his siblings would take into their work as educators.

College presented new challenges for Gerardo—challenges that he not only would overcome but that also would help shape his professional and personal commitments. Although the private liberal arts college he attended was only 50 miles from his home, he was entering an entirely new social environment, one with far greater diversity than he had ever experienced. This was where he learned what it was like to be in the minority, no longer surrounded by Latino classmates who shared similar backgrounds and experiences. And there was far greater socioeconomic diversity, too. Many of his college classmates had attended private schools, lived in spacious homes in gated communities, and traveled to places that Gerardo had seen only on television or in magazines. For the first time in his life, Gerardo learned about the dynamics of difference and power, and how race, ethnicity, gender, income, and many other factors influenced one's experience of the world. There were times that Gerardo found himself struggling to overcome feelings of doubt and uncertainty—could he succeed in this new, different culture? But, as with his earlier educational experiences, hard work and determination led to success.

Now he was ready to take the next step on his path to becoming a physician—four years of medical school. For this, Gerardo would venture far from his home in southern California, moving all the way across the country to New York, where he attended the Albert Einstein College of Medicine of Yeshiva University. Almost 3,000 miles from home, he learned what it was like to live far from family and to see them only infrequently. No longer could he look forward to weekend visits with his parents and siblings. As challenging as medical school was, Gerardo was determined to seek out experiences that would "keep him grounded." A summer trip to La Paz, Bolivia, with Child Family Health International and his volunteer work at the medical school's free clinic for the uninsured served as powerful reminders of the health disparities that exist abroad and at home, and the need to constantly work toward **health equity**.

After his four years of medical school, Gerardo—now Dr. Gerardo Lopez-Mena—made the move to Johns Hopkins and Baltimore. He immediately felt at home, but the hours would be long and the challenges of developing into a knowledgeable and skillful physician would be great. Still, he knew he wanted to do more than learn how to provide high-quality care for the patients he saw in the hospital and clinics. He wanted to reach out to the community and help people understand how to better care for themselves and how to utilize medical services in a timely and appropriate fashion. The Lay Health Educator Program offered by Johns Hopkins Bayview Medical Center was ideal for him. It gave him an opportunity to teach volunteers from local congregations about important health topics and then follow up by meeting with members of their congregations and communities who attended programs the volunteers organized. The Lay Health Educator Program also provided him with valuable insights into the everyday lives of those residing in the neighborhoods around the hospital and what was most important to them, as well as helping him learn how to communicate more effectively with his patients and their families.

Dr. Lopez-Mena was impressed by the enthusiasm of these volunteers and the impact the program was having in the community. They recognized the value of a program that focused on raising the level of **health literacy** in the community and empowering individuals to take more control over their health and health care. He also knew that the need for such a program was even greater in the Latino community, where so many spoke little or no English. This is what led him to approach the leaders of the Lay Health Educator Program to ask if he could take the initiative to develop a Spanish-language version. They quickly embraced his proposal and offered their support.

The next step was to meet with Father Robert Wojtek—or "Father Bob," as he preferred to be addressed—of Sacred Heart of Jesus Catholic Church, where large numbers of the Latino community worshipped and also gathered frequently for cultural festivals and other community events. Dr. Lopez-Mena wasn't certain at all how his proposal would be received by Father Bob. Would he see the need for such a program? Would he want the church to be involved in activities that focused primarily on physical and mental health? How would he feel about partnering with a hospital and medical professionals?

Whatever doubts or concerns Dr. Lopez-Mena had, they were quickly laid to rest. Father Bob was well aware of the health needs of his Latino parishioners. He had served for a number of years as a missionary in South America, spoke fluent Spanish, and was closely attuned to the many obstacles and challenges facing the Latino community. He understood how this program could benefit members of this community, and he felt it was consistent with his belief the church should attend to the health of its parishioners. Furthermore, he saw the value of collaborating with a medical institution in these efforts. He felt that the Latino community would be more receptive to health information and more likely to heed the recommendations of health professionals if the program was associated with the church, an institution widely viewed as safe and trustworthy. These views were expressed eloquently in later correspondence: "I have always believed that, as Church, we cannot just limit our pastoral concern to the care of souls. Those souls live in bodies, and we have responsibilities to also care for them. Thus, our approach must include the whole person. Nor can we forget that we are not alone as we seek to respond to certain needs of the whole person. So then, we must also be open to collaboration with others who can help us better serve our people."

> We cannot just limit our pastoral concern to the care of souls. Those souls live in bodies, and we have responsibilities to also care for them.

Recognizing the importance of winning the support of the congregation's lay leadership, Father Bob invited Dr. Lopez-Mena to give a presentation about the proposed program at the next meeting of the parish council. His presentation was warmly received, and he was invited to return whenever possible so they could stay informed and engaged. Then came the challenge of introducing the program to the Latino community. The first step was to give it the right name. "Lay Health Educator" didn't translate well into Spanish, so it was decided to instead call it Embajadores de Salud—Ambassadors for Health. The next step was for Father Bob to make an announcement about the health education classes during the Sunday Mass given in Spanish and invite interested individuals to join Dr. Lopez-Mena in the parish hall immediately after the worship service for lunch and more information about the program. This was an important and necessary step, but turnout was not as great as had been hoped. The same was true of the first health education class. Only a handful showed up.

Dr. Lopez-Mena admits that initially he was discouraged by the low turnout and that it would have been easy to give up, but he also cites this as one of his most valuable lessons in community building—the importance of being present, reliable, and consistent. People need to see that you are strongly committed to what you are offering and that you will be there to provide your services, even if there is only a small audience. Furthermore, Gerardo now looks at the early low turnout as a blessing in disguise because it forced him to question his whole approach. It was then that he received crucial advice from Dr. Dan Hale, his mentor and founder of the Lay Health Educator program. "I recall Dr. Hale telling me to share my personal story with the community—that it was an important story and would help the community members identify with my plight. Not only was that great advice to break the ice, but Dr. Hale's words also gave me enormous confidence that my story and our work were worth sharing." Father Bob also refused to allow himself to be discouraged. He continued to promote the program, and demonstrated his support by stopping by the classes whenever he could.

Dr. Lopez-Mena also learned that sometimes you will discover in a small group one participant who quickly "catches the vision" and becomes inspired to help you take the program to the next level. In this case, it was Monica Guerrero Vazquez, a recent arrival in Baltimore. She could see the potential for such a program and was eager to work with Dr. Lopez-Mena to make it a success. She not only assisted with the arrangements for each class but also served as a liaison with the church and community groups that offered their resources to the program. As it turns out, this was her first step on a path that would lead to her becoming the program manager for Johns Hopkins Medicine's Centro SOL (Center for Salud and Opportunities for Latinos), where she eventually would assume a major role in expanding Embajadores de Salud and other programs for the Latino community.

As Embajadores de Salud got underway, several of Dr. Lopez-Mena's colleagues in the internal medicine residency program volunteered their services, as did faculty from the Johns Hopkins University School of Medicine. Some taught classes, others helped with screenings, and still others worked with the children who often accompanied their parents to classes. Many had a long-standing interest in addressing the health needs of the Latino community, and now they had an effective way to do so. By the end of the first year, this group of community-minded health professionals had offered programs on a number of topics of importance to the Latino community, including heart disease, hypertension, diabetes, cancer, and vaccinations.

There was no question that the classes had been informative, but Monica and many of her fellow classmates in the Embajadores de Salud program realized that now they needed to take the important step of putting into practice what they had learned in their classes. For example, they now had a better understanding of how their daily routines and habits, especially what they ate, could impact their health. If they were to benefit from this knowledge, they would need to learn how to prepare meals that would be nutritious but still appeal to their families. To assist them with this, Embajadores de Salud began offering cooking classes led by a Spanish-speaking dietitian who explained how to read the nutrition information panels on the food at the grocery store and taught them how to fix meals that were both nutritious and tasty. Interest and participation in these classes grew, and soon they were holding recipe contests to see who could prepare the tastiest nutritious meals.

Course participants also had learned the important role physical activity could play in maintaining their health. They decided that the best way to increase their activity levels would be to schedule group exercise sessions so they could provide encouragement for each other and monitor their progress by regularly measuring their weight and blood pressure. Initially, they held these twice a month but soon realized it was easier to sustain their efforts if they instead met weekly. With the enthusiastic leadership of Drew White, a Johns Hopkins medical student who spoke Spanish and had a passion for exercise that was contagious, the group began meeting every Saturday—outdoors during the warm months and in the church's parish hall when the weather turned cold—and soon was attracting new members and setting ambitious goals, including running in an annual 5K run sponsored by Johns Hopkins Bayview Medical Center.

Father Bob and Monica also saw an opportunity to reach out to older adults and address some of their health concerns by inviting health professionals to attend and discuss various topics at Comiendo Juntos (Spanish for "eating together"), a monthly gathering for seniors held at the church. Organized by Monica, topics have included diabetes, stroke, dementia, **chronic kidney disease**, depression, nutrition, vaccinations, talking with your doctor and pharmacist, medication management, advance directives, and how to prevent falls.

Dr. Lopez-Mena and the other health professionals who were participating with Embajadores de Salud, as well as Father Bob, Monica, and the lay leaders at church, were pleased with what the program was accomplishing. They could see its impact, not only on the individuals who had completed the training, but also among others in the community who were hearing through their informal networks how to take better care of themselves, how to monitor their health, and when and where they should seek medical care. But it soon became apparent that there was another major health issue in the Latino community that had not yet been addressed—mental health. Father Bob was well aware of this need. Every week he had Latino parishioners coming to him for help as they and their families struggled with old and new challenges that often left them seriously depressed or highly anxious. He also would hear stories of alcohol and drug abuse. Physicians who were providing care for Latino patients also saw this need. They recognized that often the medical complaints that brought Latino patients to their offices had their roots in traumatic life experiences—some that occurred since their arrival in Baltimore and others that occurred in their home countries or on their journeys to the United States.

That many in the Latino immigrant community would be showing signs of stress is hardly surprising. Traumatic experiences were common, many dating back to their home countries, where they had lived in extreme poverty and often been the victims of, or at least witnessed, violent gang warfare. It wasn't unusual for them to know of a family member or friend who had been murdered simply because they had crossed into the "wrong" neighborhood or refused to join a gang. And escape from these situations brought new dangers and hardships. Unable to obtain visas, they often were at the mercy of dishonest coyotes (smugglers) who promised to take them across the border. Along their lengthy and physically demanding journeys, they frequently found themselves hungry and severely dehydrated, and robberies and assaults were common. Once they had made it to the United States, there were new stresses. The housing they found usually was in the poorer neighborhoods known for crime, gangs, and drug problems. Because they had entered the country illegally and thus were reluctant to have any contact with the police or other law enforcement officers, they were easy targets for crime and exploitation. And they lived every day with the fear of being discovered and detained or deported.

But providing mental health care presented serious challenges. Most of those who needed this care were unable to afford it. And even when affordable care was available, there was reluctance to take advantage of it, due largely to the stigma associated with mental illness and seeing a mental health professional. If this need was going to be addressed, it would require a different approach. What emerged was Testimonios, a community-based support group for Latino immigrants that provides a safe place for them to share their immigration experiences—to talk about what life was like in their home country, what they encountered as they made their way to the United States, and what life has been like since they arrived. These free sessions, moderated by bilingual professionals from Johns Hopkins, also give them the opportunity to develop new coping skills and strategies and to learn about community resources. The groups meet weekly, alternating between men and women, and are held at the Gallery Church, a Protestant church where many in the Latino community worship. Much like Sagrado Corazón de Jesús, the church offers services in Spanish and is known in the Latino community as a safe and welcoming congregation. The group meetings include dinner, and children who accompany their parents are offered assistance with reading and homework. And in response to the mental health needs of unaccompanied minors, there is now a Teen Testimonios program.

As the fifth anniversary of the birth of these programs passes, their continuation reinforces their importance in the community. Both Dr. Lopez-Mena and Father Bob have moved on to new positions and challenges, but the partnership endures and the programs are thriving. Dr. Lopez-Mena completed his internal medicine residency in 2014 and moved to Texas, where he now is in a leadership role at a hospital that serves a community where more than 80 percent of the population is Hispanic or Latino. In 2015, Father Bob moved to a parish in Annapolis, Maryland, where he continues a ministry that includes work with a sizable Latino community. Monica Guerrero Vazquez continues to serve as the program manager for Centro SOL, organizing Embajadores de Salud, Testimonios, Comiendo Juntos, and other programs serving the growing Latino community of Baltimore. Father Bruce Lewandowski has succeeded Father Bob at Sacred Heart of Jesus and, like his predecessor, enthusiastically supports these programs. And community participation in the programs continues to grow.

4

Medical-Religious Partnerships
and Community Health

The health ministries of Westminster By-The-Sea Presbyterian Church, Southern Baptist Church, and Sacred Heart of Jesus / Sagrado Corazón de Jesús are excellent examples of how religious congregations can effectively address serious health challenges by working in partnership with health care organizations, and there are many more such programs throughout the country. We have worked with congregations of all sizes and various faiths, some in large cities and others in suburban communities and small towns. Despite differences in size and religious beliefs and practices, these congregations share several features that make them ideal partners for health care organizations interested in reaching out into the community.

One of the most important features is that houses of worship are the only place in our society where older adults, the age group with the greatest prevalence of chronic conditions, gather regularly in large numbers. Although you may have seen or heard reports about how overall religious participation has decreased in recent decades, this decline has not been as great as sometimes thought and has occurred almost entirely among younger generations. What is often overlooked in the highly publicized (and

90 percent of adults ages 65 and older reported a religious affiliation, as did 84 percent of those in the 50- to 64-year-old age group.

cleverly titled) report, *"Nones" on the Rise: One-in-Five Adults Have No Religious Affiliation*, is that 90 percent of adults ages 65 and older reported a religious affiliation, as did 84 percent of those in the 50- to 64-year-old age group. And even among younger generations, the majority of adults still reported being religiously affiliated—77 percent of those ages 30–49 and 67 percent of young adults ages 18–29. So, in spite of some decline in religious affiliation and participation, the United States remains a highly religious country.[1]

Another important finding about religious affiliation and participation, especially given the growing diversity of the US population and our recognition of persistent health disparities among African American and Hispanic/Latino adults that must be addressed, is that regular attendance is higher among these two groups than among non-Hispanic/Latino whites. Furthermore, African American and Hispanic/Latino adults are more likely to report that religion is an important part of their daily lives, when making personal decisions, and as part of their identity.

Religious congregations bring several other important features to partnerships with health care organizations:

- One important aspect is their sheer number, with roughly 350,000 religious congregations in the United States,[2] or approximately 70 congregations for each of the country's almost 5,000 community hospitals.[3] These congregations are generally spread throughout the various neighborhoods of a community and thus are accessible and familiar to residents.

- Religious congregations are not only located in the community but also generally established and governed in large measure by residents of the community. Thus, they are likely to reflect the traditions and values of community residents and to be trusted as well.

- Most religious congregations have excellent facilities and equipment for educational programs, with ample parking and seating.

- Religious congregations generally have well-established communication networks that allow them to stay in regular contact with their members. Information can be shared by announcements during congregational gatherings, bulletins distributed at worship services, newsletters and other mailings sent to members at their home, websites, emails, social media, and volunteer phone networks.

- Perhaps most important is the **human capital** found within religious congregations. This term embraces the rich human resources within most religious institutions. Churches, synagogues, mosques, and temples have established traditions of volunteerism and civic engagement. In every congregation there are members, especially among those who are older, who are willing not only to volunteer their time but also to participate in congregational training programs that enhance their ability to step into leadership roles and to be of service to others. Many are retirees with rich experience able to bring incredible energy to a task.

Reaching beyond the Congregation

The communication networks and volunteer activities found in congregations typically reach well beyond the membership. Robert Putnam, in his acclaimed analysis of American society, *Bowling Alone: The Collapse and Revival of American Community*, describes faith communities as "arguably the single most important repository of social capital in America" (66).[4] He cites a number of studies to support this claim. For example, "In one survey of twenty-two different types of voluntary associations, from hobby groups to sports clubs to service clubs, it was membership in religious groups that was most closely associated with other forms of civic involvement, like voting, jury service, community projects, talking with neighbors, and giving to charity" (67). And he reports that "religiously involved people seem simply to know more people. One intriguing survey that asked people to enumerate all individuals with whom they had had a face-to-face conversation in the course of the day found that religious attendance was the most powerful predictor of the number of one's daily personal encounters. Regular church attendees reported talking with 40 percent more people in the course of the day" (67).

Putnam, in a later book, *American Grace: How Religion Divides and Unites Us* (coauthored by David Campbell), provides further evidence of the impact religiously active individuals have on their communities.[5] For example, the volunteerism of religious individuals usually is not limited to their congregation. In fact, there is a positive correlation between volunteering for religious groups and volunteering for secular groups. Putnam and Campbell report, "Those of us who volunteer for religious groups are two or three times as likely to volunteer for secular groups as well, compared to those of us who don't volunteer for religious groups" (445). And they found that highly religious individuals are more likely to serve as an officer or committee member of some organization, and to report that they have "worked together with others to solve a community problem" (455). They also note that religious individuals are more generous with their charitable contributions, being more likely than those not religiously affiliated to donate financially to secular causes.

Additional evidence of the potential impact religious individuals can have on their community if they become involved in health programs can be found in studies of how they are viewed by others. Their perceived trustworthiness would certainly be important when they are delivering health information to members of their community. Interestingly, Putnam and Campbell have found that "most Americans, whatever their own degree of religiosity, seem to have a trust bias in favor of religious people" (460). Even though there may be no direct evidence that religious individuals are more trustworthy than nonreligious individuals, it seems that most Americans believe they are.

These and other studies strongly suggest that if you want to initiate any new program in a community, especially one with a focus on the physical or emotional needs of the residents, faith communities are your ideal starting point. Religious congregations are where you will find individuals who have large social networks, are active in other community organizations, give generously of their time and money, and typically are viewed by others as trustworthy.

These features of religious congregations certainly indicate that they are well suited to serve as partners for health care organizations interested in improving the health of their communities, but an important question remains: How do clergy and members of religious institutions feel about devoting congregational time and resources to health programs?

To answer this question, we conducted two surveys.[6] In both cases, we were surprised by the high level of interest. In our first study, we had the opportunity to survey clergy who were attending a weeklong continuing education program. This program drew clergy from more than 20 states and a dozen denominations. It is important to note that the focus of this program was not on health ministries or any health-related topic but on preaching and theology. We developed a questionnaire titled "Partnering with Hospitals: What Do You Think?" The pastors were asked to "assume that a hospital in your community wants to work with you to enhance the health of the members of your congregation. The hospital is offering various programs and services to you at no cost, but it does ask that you support its efforts by providing leadership and assistance in certain areas."

Ninety-eight pastors completed the survey. Three-fourths of these came from five denominations (Baptist, Lutheran, Methodist, Presbyterian, and Disciples of Christ). Seventy-two percent of the respondents said that it was "very important" for churches to actively address the health needs of their congregations. The remaining 28 percent said it was "somewhat important." None of the pastors felt that it was of little or no importance.

When we asked about specific health-related offerings, we found that 80 percent or more of these clergy favored using congregational facilities for screenings (e.g., blood pressure checks), preventive interventions (e.g., flu vaccinations), and health-related classes (e.g., nutrition, stress management). Eighty percent also said they would offer support for volunteers in their congregations trained to provide assistance for congregational members who needed help at home or when they visited their physician. Two-thirds of the clergy reported that they favored using congregational mailings or newsletters to announce the availability of screenings designed to detect serious medical conditions (e.g., hypertension, diabetes) and that they would personally encourage their congregation to participate in regular screenings.

We then surveyed more than 500 members of religious congregations. Two-thirds of these respondents came from five religious groups: Baptist, Methodist, Presbyterian, Catholic, and Lutheran. A brief paragraph at the top of their questionnaire stated, "Many hospitals and medical professionals would like to help churches (synagogues) address the health needs and concerns of their members. We would like to know if church (synagogue) members are interested in having health programs in their church (synagogue)."

Eighty-five percent reported that they would like to have educational programs on health matters presented at their church or synagogue, and 45 percent indicated they would be interested in helping organize or promote these health programs. The top choices for programs were:

- Stress management
- Alzheimer's disease (or other forms of dementia)
- Cancer
- Heart disease
- Depression
- Cardiopulmonary resuscitation
- **Living wills**, do not resuscitate orders, and other advance directives
- Arthritis
- Diabetes
- Healthy meal preparation
- Hypertension
- Stroke

When we asked about other types of health-related programs or concerns, we found that three-quarters wanted health screenings (e.g., blood pressure, blood sugar, cholesterol, or skin cancer) and preventive measures (e.g., flu vaccinations) to be available at church. Four out of five respondents thought there were people in their congregation who needed more exercise and would be interested in joining a walking group or other exercise group that met regularly at their church (55 percent reported they would be interested in participating in such a program). A similar number thought there were individuals in their church who may be depressed but were not getting the treatment or help they needed and that there were individuals in their church who would benefit from being a member of a support group that meets regularly.

These surveys indicate strong support among clergy and laity for congregational health programs. Further evidence of the high level of support for congregational health programs comes from another survey. The Baylor Religion Survey (2005), a nationally representative survey of 1,721 respondents that included nearly 400 items, provided an extensive and in-depth analysis of the religious beliefs and practices of Americans.[7] One of the interesting findings of this study was that the most commonly held value among their respondents was taking care of the sick and needy. This ranked higher than teaching others your morals, converting others to your religious faith, or any of the other options. And this high level of support for taking care of the sick and needy cut across all religious and theological divisions.

Preventive Medicine

How can congregations merge their interests in health matters with the resources of health care organizations to produce effective health programs? Although health concerns will vary from congregation to congregation, we have found the best way to begin planning for and organizing health programs is to adopt the basic principles and methods of preventive medicine. This field is dedicated to keeping people healthy and preventing, or at least greatly reducing, the risk of premature illness, disability, and death. The key to effective preventive medicine programs is getting medical information and resources to people in a timely and easy-to-understand, easy-to-use fashion. The goal is to have everyone acquire a better understanding of what can be done to maintain their health, independence, and dignity. In the remainder of this chapter, we review the basic concepts of preventive medicine and illustrate how these can be incorporated into the life and mission of religious congregations.

Preventive practices and interventions are generally organized into three categories or levels: primary, secondary, and tertiary. The following sections provide descriptions and examples of programs at each of these levels.

Primary Prevention

The goal of **primary prevention** is to prevent the development of disease or disability. By engaging in health-enhancing practices and avoiding or minimizing health-compromising activities, people can greatly reduce their risk of developing various chronic conditions and experiencing serious injuries. Included in this category are both lifestyle modifications and immunizations. Some examples are giving up smoking, exercising regularly, eating nutritious meals, preventing injuries, and obtaining vaccinations against influenza, pneumonia, shingles, and tetanus.

Since most of us would put good health at or near the top of our list of personal goals, it seems like it should be fairly easy to persuade people to adopt health-enhancing practices and cut back on any health-compromising activities. But much of the time it actually can be quite difficult. Too often people do not pay attention to health matters until a serious illness or injury strikes. And this is understandable. If they are feeling fine doing what they have always been doing, they may see no reason to make any changes in their habits and routines, especially when there are no immediate benefits. Even when individuals believe that ignoring such advice may have negative consequences on their health, the changes they need to make now may seem too costly because the harmful consequences of their behavior may not occur until much later in their lives.

Religious institutions have certain advantages when sponsoring primary prevention programs. First, they can incorporate information about primary prevention practices into regularly scheduled programs. In this way, they have a "built-in" audience. Second, they can present the information in different formats and at various times. This is important because one message alone is seldom sufficient to produce lasting changes in long-standing behavior patterns. Repetition and reinforcement are almost always required. Third, most religious congregations have members of all ages. This allows them to schedule intergenerational programs on health matters. They can encourage older adults, especially those who have developed chronic illnesses, to bring their children and even grandchildren to an informational program. Children and grandchildren are more likely to listen to and heed the advice on illness prevention measures when they can see firsthand the impact chronic diseases could have on their lives.

Example of a Congregational Primary Prevention Program

A simple and yet effective primary prevention initiative you can sponsor for your congregation is one that encourages members, and especially older adults, to get annual influenza vaccinations. The Centers for Disease Control and Prevention reports that even though some years there have been as many as 56,000 flu-related deaths and 710,000 flu-related hospitalizations, less than half of all adults take advantage of flu vaccinations.[8] This is an especially serious matter for older adults, the age group at greatest risk of serious complications of the flu, with an estimated 71–85 percent of flu-related deaths occurring in people 65 years and older.[9] It is also important to note that vaccination rates are lower among African Americans and other racial and ethnic groups than non-Hispanic/Latino whites, reflecting a pattern of health disparity seen in other measures of preventive health in the United States.[10] In spite of the grave dangers associated with influenza and substantial evidence for the effectiveness of the vaccine, large numbers of older adults fail to get annual vaccinations. Education programs sponsored jointly by congregations and respected health organizations can increase the number of vaccinations and decrease the number of hospitalizations and deaths due to influenza. Participation can be increased even more by arranging for the health department or a hospital to offer vaccinations after the worship service or other well-attended congregational programs. This is what Baltimore's Southern Baptist Church arranged. The program included having a physician speak briefly about flu and the importance of vaccinations during the worship service. Then, at the conclusion of the service, the pastor, Dr. Donté Hickman, encouraged congregants to follow him to the fellowship hall, where they would be able to get flu vaccinations provided by the Baltimore City Health Department.

> **Some years there have been as many as 56,000 flu-related deaths and 710,000 flu-related hospitalizations.**

Secondary Prevention

The goal of **secondary prevention** is to detect a disease in its earliest stages in order to cure it or slow its progression. Screening tests can identify some medical conditions (e.g., diabetes, hypertension) before symptoms become evident. Once a diagnosis is made, treatment can begin and the progression of the disease and its complications may be slowed or even prevented. In this way, the development of disability can be slowed and life can even be prolonged. Once a disease or condition has been detected, interventions may include either strictly medical measures or some of the lifestyle modifications listed in the section on primary prevention. Recommended screenings generally include breast cancer, colorectal cancer, skin cancer, hypertension (high blood pressure), **hyperlipidemia**, diabetes, HIV/AIDS, and depression and potential for suicide.

Time and transportation can be barriers to secondary prevention. Many people complain that they do not have the time in their busy schedules to participate in medical screenings and counseling, particularly when they are feeling healthy. Other individuals, especially many older adults, may have the time for screenings but find it difficult to arrange transportation. Religious congregations can help overcome both of these barriers by arranging screenings to be conducted on-site and in conjunction with regularly scheduled congregational gatherings. Hospitals, home health agencies, city or county health departments, nurses, and physicians can be enlisted to assist in these screenings. If you cannot arrange to have screenings conducted in your congregational facilities, you still can facilitate the screenings by arranging for transportation to and from the local hospital, health department, or medical laboratory.

Examples of Congregational Secondary Prevention Programs

An excellent example of a secondary prevention program is the skin cancer screening that is a regular event at Westminster By-The-Sea Presbyterian Church. The high level of participation in this valuable program is the result of reliable information about skin cancer, the strong endorsement of Dr. Sumner, the church's pastor, and the fact that the screenings are conducted immediately after the Sunday worship service.

Another simple, inexpensive secondary prevention program that can be sponsored by a religious congregation is one in which volunteer nurses, other health care professionals, or properly trained volunteers provide blood pressure checks before or after the worship service. Little time and equipment are required for this program, but it can yield highly meaningful results. By identifying people with high blood pressure and encouraging them to take appropriate measures to bring their blood pressure under control, you can reduce the **incidence** of heart attacks and strokes. Announcements in congregational bulletins and from respected congregational leaders can increase the number of people participating in and benefiting from this program.

Tertiary Prevention

The goal of **tertiary prevention** is to reduce the complications and disabilities associated with an existing disease. This often is referred to by health professionals as disease or illness management. Most of the responsibility for illness management falls on patients and their families, so it is important for all those affected to learn how to manage chronic medical conditions effectively. Good management can help persons live longer and, ideally, also maintain their independence and a good quality of life. Some preventive measures at the tertiary level are:

- Identifying and using appropriate medical services in a timely fashion
- Taking medications correctly
- Using community resources to enhance functional health
- Participating in support groups for patients, family members, and caregivers in order to improve coping, strengthen resilience, and avoid despondency and burnout

Religious congregations provide ideal venues for numerous types of tertiary prevention programs. Many people who have chronic conditions fail to receive appropriate treatments and related services because they do not know about various medical and community resources, or they have encountered obstacles when trying to access services. Within congregations, there are usually clergy or lay leaders who are aware of many community medical services and other community agencies, often serving in leadership positions in these organizations. They can compile and pass along the information about community resources to members who need these services, and some may want to offer to serve as advocates on behalf of those having difficulty obtaining services. Also, to ensure that members who live alone are doing well, many congregations have programs in which volunteers regularly check on them by telephone. These volunteers can also be easily trained to use these contacts to remind members about their medication or appointments. Support groups for patients or families also fit well within the mission and ministry of most congregations and can provide the encouragement patients and families affected by a chronic condition often need.

Examples of Congregational Tertiary Prevention Programs

One way a congregation can assist in tertiary prevention (or disease management) is to sponsor a support group for people with a specific condition or for their families experiencing disease-related stress. These groups can be helpful in many ways. Some people find it difficult to follow through with their treatment regimens on a consistent basis once the crisis seems to have passed. For example, some patients with heart disease will revert back to unhealthy dietary practices or abandon regular exercise programs once they feel they have recovered from a heart attack. Support groups can give these people and their families and caregivers the assistance and support they need to maintain their new regimens. Support groups also can help patients and their loved ones cope with some of the limitations and emotional aspects of an illness. Often new coping strategies can be learned from other members of the group.

The programs on medication management, particularly the ones addressing cholesterol-lowering medications, are another good example of a simple yet important approach to tertiary prevention. A common mistake made by individuals taking cholesterol-lowering medications is that, once their cholesterol levels have reached the desired range, they believe they do not need to continue taking the medication. Having pharmacists and physicians explain how these medications work and the need for people to continue taking them after their cholesterol levels have reached the target levels—unless their physicians instruct them to discontinue the medication—can reduce the risk of heart attack.

5

Congregational Health
Education Programs

One of the most valuable and meaningful programs that can be offered to a congregation and community is a proactive health education program. Information is at the heart of both health promotion and illness management. People of all ages, even children, need to know more about health, illnesses, and medical care. Most of the life-limiting and life-threatening diseases encountered in middle or late adulthood have their roots in earlier years. Members of your congregation and community need clear, reliable information about steps they can take to promote wellness and reduce the risks of developing illnesses. Congregants who already have medical conditions need reliable, easy-to-understand information about how they can effectively manage their conditions, reduce the likelihood of developing disability, and even prolong life.

The importance of providing people with information they can understand and act on arises from research on health literacy. The Institute of Medicine, in its report, *Health Literacy: A Prescription to End Confusion* (2004),[1] defines health literacy as "the degree to which individuals have the capacity to obtain, communicate, process, and understand basic health information and services in order to make appropriate health decisions." The impact health literacy has on health is illustrated in the findings of an extensive review of the literature on health literacy and health outcomes[2] that found, "Low health literacy was consistently associated with:

- more hospitalizations;
- greater use of emergency care;
- lower receipt of mammography screening and influenza vaccine;

While it might strike some people as surprising for churches and other faith communities to include providing health education as part of their mission, there are interesting historical precedents. During the eighteenth century, when there was no universal, compulsory education and many children were forced to work six days a week in factories, religious philanthropists in Great Britain, eager to give these children the opportunity for a better life, came up with an innovative solution.[3] Why not use Sundays, the one day children were not in the factories, to teach them to read and write? And why not make this education available in churches? This movement soon spread to the United States, with denominational and nondenominational organizations creating programs for children who otherwise would not receive a basic education. Thus, Sunday schools were born. Not for religious instruction, but to address the problem of illiteracy.

Sunday schools played an especially important role in addressing basic literacy for African Americans in the southern states during and after the Civil War.[4] These schools, often referred to as Sabbath or Midnight schools, were sponsored by churches and offered classes in the evenings and on weekends for individuals who were unable to attend weekday classes. That these schools emphasized more than biblical or religious lessons can be seen in Booker T. Washington's report of his own experience, noting that "the principal book studied in the Sunday school was the spelling book."[5]

- poorer ability to demonstrate taking medications appropriately;
- poorer ability to interpret labels and health messages;
- and, among elderly persons, poorer overall health status and higher mortality rates."

Additionally, it was found that some racial disparities are explained in part by health literacy.

Addressing Health Literacy in the Congregation

Physicians, psychologists, and other researchers in the field of preventive medicine have developed a large body of scientific information about the steps people can take to prevent illnesses or at least lessen their impact. There is reliable information about the activities or practices that increase the odds of staying healthy as well as those that increase the odds of developing chronic illnesses. There are also well-established methods for detecting many diseases in the early stages, thus limiting their harmful effects.

Most of this information about health promotion, early detection programs, and illness
management is straightforward and easy for
people to understand. You do not need to possess in-depth knowledge about the biological or
medical aspects of most illnesses to understand what types of activity will enhance your health and what types may compromise your health. Nor do you have to understand exactly how medical examinations are analyzed to receive the benefits of regular monitoring of certain key measures of your health.

Some racial disparities are explained in part by health literacy.

Although most of the information we need about health matters is easy to understand, too many of us fail to take advantage of it. Either we do not seek out the necessary information, even when it is readily available, or we fail to act on it. Why? The reasons vary from person to person, and we need to understand and be sensitive to these reasons as we plan and implement a health education program. We need to invite individuals to tell us about their lives and their health concerns and listen carefully when they do.

Overcoming Barriers to Wellness Promotion

Some people simply are not motivated to seek out information on health matters until a medical crisis arises. As long as they feel well, they are not interested in reading materials or attending programs on health issues. These individuals either are not aware of or not concerned about the eventual consequences of their health-compromising actions. In fact, studies have found that although health is generally ranked at or near the top of values people hold, somewhere between 20 and 40 percent of people do not rank it in their top five.[6]

Some individuals say they ignore information on health matters because they are confused by the various warnings and recommendations, which often seem contradictory, and they do not know what to believe. Others believe the information they have heard is reliable, but they are not motivated to act on it. They know that modifying some aspects of their lifestyle would be beneficial, but they cannot seem to make the necessary changes. Sometimes they are too busy with other pressing responsibilities to focus on their health. Other people know what course of action they should take and make a decision to follow up on it but then have difficulty staying on track. This is not surprising, because most of us find it hard to make lasting changes unless we receive regular reminders and ongoing encouragement and support.

Whatever the reasons, too many people fail to use valuable information on health to their advantage. In fact, one of the greatest challenges in health care is finding an effective means of delivering health information directly to the people who need it most, persuading them that they will benefit from this information, and providing the ongoing support they need to faithfully adhere to well-established prevention and treatment regimens. The challenge is to find innovative and appealing ways of reaching people.

Religious institutions, through their professional and lay leaders, can play a crucial role in bringing information and people together. Congregational leaders have the opportunity and ability to reach people *before* they encounter a medical crisis. Furthermore, they can present the information in ways that can be understood and appreciated by the members of their congregations and communities, and they can design informational programs that overcome many of the obstacles encountered in most community health education programs. These leaders have the potential to empower people by giving them the knowledge and tools to maintain their health and independence.

Although congregational leaders have many tangible and intangible resources that they can use in their efforts to minister to the health needs of their congregations, they still face significant challenges. Effective health education programs require a multifaceted, proactive approach. You have to do more than simply place attractive brochures in the pews or hold occasional health fairs.

First, you must get people's attention. You have to find ways for the information you are providing to stand out from everything else people are reading and hearing. This is not always an easy task, especially when many of us find ourselves experiencing information overload almost every day, but somehow you must reach out to people and convince them that you have information they need to hear. Second, you need to persuade them that there are decisions they can make and actions they can take that will yield personal health benefits. Third, you must convince them that the benefits of their decisions and actions outweigh the costs. Fourth, you need to bring them together in support of each other as they work to adopt and maintain health-enhancing actions.

The Health Belief Model

We have found the most helpful model to use in planning is the health belief model.[7] This simple model, widely used throughout the health care field, can help you organize the presentation of information such that it will have the greatest impact on your audiences. The four components of this model are presented below, followed by an example that applies the health belief model to hypertension.

First, you must convince people that they are susceptible to a disease or condition. They need to understand that they—or their loved ones—could already have or eventually develop the disease or condition that is being discussed. People who are unaware that they are vulnerable to a particular disease (e.g., diabetes, hypertension, glaucoma) are not likely to take the correct steps to prevent its onset or detect it in the earliest stages.

Second, you need to persuade people that the disease or condition can have severe consequences. It is not enough for people to believe that they are susceptible to an illness; they must also realize that it can be seriously harmful. They must see that a particular disease or condition could greatly limit their ability to enjoy their favorite activities or even shorten their life. People who believe that they may be susceptible to a particular illness but do not believe that the illness can have serious consequences ("Yes, I have high blood pressure, but it's not a big deal") are unlikely to make any significant modifications in their lifestyle or health practices.

Third, people must believe in the efficacy or power of the prevention or treatment recommendations. You need to convince people that there are steps they can take that will reduce the risk of becoming ill or minimize the impact of a disease. If people believe that there are no effective treatments for a disease ("There's really nothing anyone can do about my condition"), they will see no reason to participate in early detection or treatment programs.

Fourth, people must believe that the benefits of illness prevention and treatment regimens outweigh the costs or burdens of those regimens. This point is often overlooked by health workers, who may not be aware of the personal costs or burdens associated with certain actions. Although the benefits may seem obvious to health care professionals, many people feel that the costs associated with various treatments outweigh the benefits. Even seemingly small costs—time away from work, transportation getting to and from appointments—may be the primary reason that elderly or low-income persons do not seek services. This is where the feedback you receive from members of your congregation and community can be helpful in identifying barriers and finding ways to overcome them. Working together, health care organizations and religious congregations may be able to find creative ways to reduce the costs or burdens associated with certain services. For example, they may be able to arrange for diabetes screenings and nutritional counseling to be offered in congregational facilities and at convenient times.

One additional variable that can be important is an instigating event or cue to action. This could be a local or national public awareness campaign (e.g., American Heart Month every February or Breast Cancer Awareness Month every October) or the testimony of a person who benefited by taking the recommended action (e.g., receiving successful treatment for a medical condition detected through a health screening). These could present you with an opportunity to build on existing awareness and interest.

Health education programs that are designed with these objectives in mind are most likely to have an impact on members of your congregation and community.

Hypertension, or high blood pressure, can illustrate how the health belief model can be used to organize educational programs. Many people are unaware of the problem of high blood pressure or do not know they are susceptible to it. Some people believe they are in good health—free of any disease as long as they do not have any painful symptoms or physical limitations. They do not think they need to concern themselves with getting their blood pressure checked unless they begin to feel ill. Therefore, the first step in educating them and helping them change their health practices is to find some way to convince them that they are susceptible to hypertension, even if they are not feeling ill or experiencing high levels of stress.

One way to help people understand that they are susceptible to hypertension is to give them information about its widespread prevalence—that it is, in fact, a very common condition. Once they realize that millions of people have hypertension but are unaware of their condition, they may be more willing to acknowledge the possibility that they, too, could have high blood pressure. This type of information also may help catch the attention of specific groups of people who are known to have high rates of hypertension (e.g., older adults, African Americans). Another way to reach and influence people is to share examples of people similar to them who discovered they had high blood pressure. (Of course, this would be done only with their permission.) Often a few such personal examples are more effective than statistics. When possible, it is best to use a combination of these two approaches because some people respond best to statistical information, while others respond best to personal stories.

Second, you need to persuade people that there are potentially severe consequences associated with hypertension. Individuals who are aware of the problem of hypertension but believe there are no serious effects associated with it are not likely to monitor their blood pressure regularly and seek treatment should it be too high. They may view it as a condition that has little significance for their overall health. Other people may attempt to dismiss the risks associated with hypertension by saying, "I have to die of something." Often this is a way of avoiding a threatening subject, but such a statement also indicates that they are overlooking serious consequences other than death. That is why it is important to remind people that high blood pressure increases their risk of heart attack and stroke, both of which may leave them seriously disabled. Although they may survive, they could be left in a condition in which they are unable to participate in many of the activities they enjoy and find rewarding. The prospect of a long-term disability is often viewed as a more undesirable outcome than death.

Third, once you have helped people understand that they are susceptible to hypertension and that it can have severe consequences, you need to persuade them that there are things they can do to help themselves. You need to offer hope and educate people about the steps to take to reduce the risk of hypertension and its potentially harmful consequences. They need to hear from reliable, trusted sources that by making certain lifestyle modifications or taking medication, they can bring their blood pressure under control.

Fourth, you must be sensitive to people's perceptions about the cost of following the recommended prevention, monitoring, and treatment regimens for hypertension. Some people may believe the financial costs of treatment outweigh the benefits, especially if they are on a limited budget and have other financial obligations. Others may fear that the side effects of the medication for their blood pressure will actually produce a poorer quality of life. Sometimes the fears about the costs or negative effects of treatment are based on erroneous beliefs that can be corrected by providing accurate information from an authoritative source. However, in some situations, costs can be a real factor. In such cases, you may be able to give information about professionals or agencies that can provide less costly treatments or offer financial assistance.

The cues to action for a congregational program on hypertension could begin with a bulletin insert with basic information on hypertension—its prevalence, the potentially harmful consequences if not treated, and treatment options. This material could be offered any time during the year, but you may want to make a special effort during either February (American Heart Month) or May (National Stroke Awareness Month), when there are public awareness campaigns in your community that would be encouraging people to learn more about hypertension. This information could be supplemented by a brief presentation by a member of the congregation who discovered through a health screening that, in spite of feeling healthy, he or she had hypertension. Finally, to overcome any time or transportation barriers, blood pressure checks could be provided immediately before or after a congregational gathering.

Employing the "Teach-Back" Method

It is not unusual for patients, when asked by their health care providers if they understand the information they have just been given on an important health matter, to answer "yes," even if they do not fully comprehend what they have been told. Because this happens so often, many health care providers now employ what is known as the "teach-back" method. In this method, providers ask patients to explain back—in their own words—what they have just learned about their condition and/or the steps they should take to treat their condition. We have found it helpful to use this method in our health education programs, whether with an individual or in a group setting. This will allow you to determine if the information has been understood correctly and, if not, you will have an opportunity to explain it again, perhaps using terminology better suited to your audience.

Motivating People to Take Action

The health belief model can be useful in designing programs and materials for your congregation. It should help as you select topics and decide what type of information needs to be presented to your congregation or community. However, although many members of your congregation will appreciate your work, your efforts may not be warmly received or appreciated by all. You may encounter resistance or criticism from others in the congregation. Some individuals may feel that you are being critical or judgmental when you encourage them to make changes in their lifestyle ("I don't come to church to be told that I need to exercise more or eat more nutritious meals"). Often people who have the greatest need to adopt new practices are the most difficult to reach. It takes a sensitive and diplomatic approach in the presentation of information to overcome this resistance. Even those who are aware that they need to alter their lifestyle or behavioral patterns often have mixed feelings about change. Yes, they genuinely want to be healthy and know that they would benefit from the recommended changes, but they also realize that by making these changes they would be giving up certain activities or habits they enjoy. Therefore, it is a good idea to know some basic principles and strategies that can be used when you are encouraging people to adopt new health practices and to abandon, or at least modify, some long-standing habits.

Two books on motivational interviewing—*Motivational Interviewing: Preparing People for Change*, by Miller and Rollnick,[8] and *Motivational Interviewing in Health Care*, by Rollnick, Miller, and Butler[9]—provide a good model appropriate for work in congregations. Although the principles and strategies they offer are generally used by health professionals working on a one-to-one basis, they also are appropriate for working with groups of people who need encouragement as they seek to incorporate health-enhancing practices into their lifestyle and discard or reduce health-compromising habits.

The first principle of motivational interviewing is to *express empathy*—letting people know you have a good understanding of how they feel about the issue you are discussing. People are more open to change when they sense that you understand—or at least are making a sincere effort to understand—their situation and the stresses and challenges they face in their life. They are more likely to listen to you and accept the information you are offering if they can tell that you know how they feel. The steps you or your speakers recommend may seem both obvious and simple to you but may strike some people as overwhelming, at least given their current circumstances. To be truly empathic, it is necessary to listen carefully and with an open mind when these individuals express their feelings and concerns about what is being recommended. You need to be willing to put yourself in their position and be able to view life from their perspective. This does not mean that you must agree with everything they say, but it does mean that you need to convey to them that you accept their actions, thoughts, and feelings without judging or criticizing them.

The second principle is to *develop discrepancy*. Although listening carefully and empathizing with people is an important and usually necessary first step in helping them to change, it is often not sufficient. For people to become motivated to actually make changes, they need to recognize that there is a discrepancy—a gap—between where they are now with respect to health-enhancing practices and where they could be. They need to understand that they will fail to achieve some worthwhile goals if they continue their current practices. The awareness of this discrepancy is what can provide the fuel or energy for change. But it is important that this perceived discrepancy be between their current state and *their* goals, not yours. They need to see the connection between the things in life they care about and their health behaviors. Therefore, you can be helpful by aiding them in identifying some goals that they truly value. These goals can vary tremendously. For some individuals, the goal of being able to live longer than their parents or with fewer health-related limitations may be best, whereas for others the goal of being able to enjoy activities with their grandchildren may be the most important.

The third principle is to *avoid argumentation*. When people feel they are being directly attacked or criticized for "bad habits" or "problem behaviors," they are likely to become defensive and develop arguments that they believe justify their current practices. Even arguing that someone *should* have a particular goal or *should* follow certain practices can lead to resistance. Instead, keep the emphasis on the positive—the benefits of adopting some of the recommendations about how to become healthier. The objective of a good health education program is not to make people feel bad about their current health status but to inspire people to become healthier. You want to help people find their own reasons for avoiding health-compromising activities and adopting health-enhancing practices.

The fourth principle is to *roll with resistance*. Do not be surprised when people seem to ignore the information and services you are offering them. Not everyone is going to appreciate what you are trying to accomplish. But do not give up. Be flexible. Approach the topic from a different perspective, or focus on another topic. If people object to your approach or seem uninterested, ask them what type of information they want or what format for health education programs is the most appealing. Listen to their feedback and involve them in your planning process. In most situations, your audience can give you helpful advice about how to approach them.

The fifth principle is to *support self-efficacy*. People need to develop the belief that they have the capacity, the power, to make changes. It is important

for them to see that they can be successful in making constructive modifications in their life. Successful experiences, even small successes, can help
people build this sense of self-efficacy. Therefore, it is helpful to encourage
people to set reasonable goals for themselves. People with sedentary life-
styles do not have to join the local gym and become great athletes; they
simply need to increase their physical activities. Any increase—even just an
additional 10–15 minutes of physical activity each day—should be viewed as
a success. Similarly, people who have become accustomed to a diet high in fat
do not have to adopt a strict low-fat diet to be successful; they need only to
reduce some of the fat in their diet to rightfully claim success. Movement in
the right direction, even if it comes in small steps, can build confidence and
raise expectations about their ability to make additional changes.

On-Site Services and Supportive Follow-Up

When planning health programs for your congregation or community,
recognize the value of on-site services. Some of the steps you or your guest
speakers are recommending may seem too costly financially or in terms of
time if people have to leave work or make special travel arrangements. For
example, some individuals may be persuaded that it would be wise for them
to monitor their blood pressure on a regular basis, but they find it difficult
to get to their doctor's office or a clinic. Problems with transportation or
scheduling may prevent them from regular visits. An easy solution to these
problems is to arrange for nurses or properly trained volunteers to provide
blood pressure checks once every month or two immediately after a worship
service or a regularly scheduled congregational meeting. Providing on-site
services will lessen the cost or burden of following the health-enhancing recommendations people have received in your educational programs. Anything
you can do to remove or reduce barriers will increase the chances of people
engaging in health-enhancing activities.

Finally, the value of regular reminders and supportive follow-up services
cannot be emphasized enough. People are not always ready for the information you are offering at the time you are offering it. For example, many
individuals may not think they need to know much about depression the first
time you provide information on mood disorders in a congregational program, because it does not seem to be a factor in their life or the lives of their
loved ones. However, a few months later they may be ready to hear about

the topic because a family member or friend is showing signs of depression. Another reason to incorporate regular messages and reminders is that most people find it difficult to make lasting changes in their behavior patterns and health practices. Friendly reminders can help them stay on track and maintain their motivation.

II SUGGESTED TOPICS FOR CONGREGATIONAL PROGRAMS

6

Coronary Artery Disease

Coronary artery disease (also known as coronary heart disease) is the most common type of heart disease and is the leading cause of death in both men and women in the United States. Each year, more than 700,000 Americans suffer a heart attack (**myocardial infarction**).[1, 2] Heart attacks occur when arterial (blood vessel) blockages stop blood and oxygen from reaching the heart muscle—as when a clogged fuel line stops a car engine. The blockage of the coronary arteries is commonly due to **atherosclerosis**, or a buildup of plaque in the arteries. The process of plaque building up and causing a thickening and narrowing of the arteries begins long before a heart attack occurs. In fact, it is a gradual process that may start as early as childhood. It is increasingly recognized that some heart attacks occur due to rupture of atherosclerotic plaques—even those that before rupturing do not obstruct the flow of blood through the affected artery. When a plaque ruptures, the rapid formation of a clot occurs and the artery can become completely blocked. Whatever the underlying physiology, rapid medical treatment in a hospital with "clot busting" drugs and interventions (such as an angioplasty, where a balloon catheter is used to open the clogged coronary artery and place a stent to keep the artery open) not only saves lives but also lessens the heart muscle damage that follows the event.

Coronary artery disease is also the leading cause of **heart failure**, a condition where the heart does not pump blood effectively. Heart failure can develop after a heart attack as heart muscle becomes injured; scar tissue replaces functional muscle; and the main heart chamber, or left ventricle, is thereby weakened and less able to pump blood forward. Over time, the weakened heart will struggle to keep up with normal demands of the body in regard to blood flow and oxygen delivery. While coronary artery disease is the most common cause for heart failure, other conditions, such as high blood pressure, faulty heart valves, and abnormal heart rhythms, can cause heart failure. All of these conditions require ongoing monitoring and medical care.

Who Is at Risk?

Risk factors for coronary artery disease fall into two groups—**modifiable** (risk factors one can modify and control) and **nonmodifiable** (risk factors one cannot control). Nonmodifiable risk factors include a person's age, gender, and family history. Of all known risk factors, older age is the most potent risk factor for coronary artery disease, since the arteries of older adults have been exposed to the other risk factors (e.g., high cholesterol, hypertension, and smoking) for a longer period of time. Further, the incidence of hypertension and diabetes, two common late-life conditions among people in the United States, increases dramatically among older age groups and may further accelerate the worsening of coronary artery disease. In addition, older adults are more vulnerable to heart disease and regularly have more complications and worse outcomes as compared to younger patients. Therefore, knowledge of the risk and early recognition and treatment of coronary artery disease are especially important among older people.

Coronary artery disease is more common in men than in women during early and middle adulthood.[1, 2] However, the risk of heart disease rises dramatically in postmenopausal women after the age of 50. Although many women fear breast cancer as the number one cause of death, heart disease affects and kills more women than all forms of cancer combined. For both men and women, heredity plays an important role because the risk of heart disease is greater for those with a family history of premature heart attacks. For individuals who do not know their family history, establishing a family health record by questioning relatives is recommended. High levels of blood cholesterol can also run in families, and many medical studies now support the identification and treatment of high cholesterol as an effective strategy in the prevention and treatment of coronary artery disease—even for adolescents and young adults.

> **Although many women fear breast cancer as the number one cause of death, heart disease affects and kills more women than all forms of cancer combined.**

One of the most common risks for coronary artery disease, particularly in older adults, is hypertension, or high blood pressure.[1] As we age, our arteries naturally get stiffer. Thus, hypertension often develops after the age of 50, even among those with good exercise and nutritional habits. Women develop hypertension with aging but about a decade later than men. Interestingly, more than 70 percent of 70-year-olds and 80 percent of 80-year-olds have high blood pressure. The type of hypertension that develops in older age is different from hypertension that develops at younger ages and is far more risky. Treating hypertension associated with aging markedly reduces the risk of coronary artery disease, heart failure, heart attacks, and other diseases (stroke, kidney disease, and dementia). Therefore, it is important to have blood pressure checked regularly to avoid or lessen the risk of developing these conditions.

Diabetes is another potent predictor of future heart disease. Because **obesity** is a significant risk factor for diabetes (and hypertension), being overweight or obese is an important risk factor for coronary artery disease as well. (To determine if individuals are overweight or obese, health care professionals generally use the **body mass index**.) In combination, diabetes, high blood pressure, and obesity are recognized by physicians as the **metabolic syndrome**. One of the simplest predictors of this syndrome is the measurement of waist size. Waist sizes greater than 40 inches for men and 35 inches for women are highly predictive of development of metabolic syndrome and the ultimate development of adverse health outcomes. Therefore, programs that address maintenance of a healthy weight and identify and control blood glucose levels and diabetes are particularly important for preventing and treating coronary artery disease.

Finally, smoking is a very significant risk factor for heart disease, and stopping smoking is the single most potent modifiable risk factor for delaying the onset of coronary artery disease. Therefore, strategies to help people stop smoking should be a priority for all communities.

The Risks of Ignoring Information on Coronary Artery Disease

The most serious and feared consequence of failing to understand and act on information about coronary artery disease is a fatal heart attack. In the United States, every 34 seconds someone has a heart attack, and every 60 seconds someone dies from a heart attack. Surviving a heart attack, though, can still have serious and long-lasting consequences, since the heart's muscle has been damaged from the heart attack.[1,2] Damaged heart muscle may lead to heart failure, with the heart too weak to pump enough blood forward to provide the body with the oxygen it needs to meet the demands of normal activities. Thus, heart failure usually results in limitations to one's day-to-day life due to excessive fatigue and weakness and is a leading cause of hospitalizations among older adults, often due to shortness of breath.

What Can Be Done to Prevent Coronary Artery Disease?

Reducing the Risk

Many steps can be taken to avoid, or at least greatly delay, the harmful consequences of heart disease. The most important ones that are within one's control include changes in lifestyle:

- *Stop smoking.* Smoking contributes to the buildup of plaque, which leads to coronary artery disease and heart attacks. While quitting smoking can be a struggle, the benefits of stopping are significant. Quitting at any age greatly improves health and reduces the risk of coronary artery disease.
- *Monitor what you eat.* Knowing how to read food labels is vital to understanding what one is eating. Recognizing that there are different types of fat and avoiding or limiting items high in saturated fat can help improve your cholesterol.
- *Exercise more often.* You do not have to join a gym or embark on a rigorous exercise program, but it is important to exercise regularly. Walking for 20–30 minutes a day is optimal. It is always advisable to discuss with your physician how much exercise is appropriate and if you qualify for formal exercise programs that are often disease-specific (e.g., cardiac rehabilitation).
- *Lose weight.* If you are overweight, lose weight by participating in a safe, gradual weight reduction program. Maintaining a healthy, stable weight is then accomplished by continuing those healthy lifestyle changes.
- *Have regular check-ups.* Many of the conditions that can lead to coronary artery disease, such as diabetes, hypertension, and hyperlipidemia, develop without any signs or symptoms. Therefore, regular checkups can screen for elevated blood pressure, and blood work can be

evaluated for glucose and cholesterol levels. Your health care provider can interpret these results and, if necessary, work with you to develop the treatment plan that will be best for you.

Detecting the Early Signs of Coronary Artery Disease

Detecting coronary artery disease can be difficult because the athero-sclerotic process is silent for the majority of time before it creates noticeable symptoms. For example, the pain and discomfort of coronary artery disease may not be experienced until 75 percent or more of the coronary artery is narrowed.[2] Chest pain due to narrowed coronary arteries is called **angina pectoris**. This chest pain results from heart muscle demanding blood and oxygen, but the coronary artery is unable to meet the demand because of the narrowing from the plaque buildup. This mismatch in supply and demand caused by the diseased coronary arteries results in ischemia (low oxygen delivery) to the heart muscle. Angina usually occurs during activity and re-solves with rest. Other symptoms of ischemia besides chest pain can include shortness of breath, nausea, cold sweats, dizziness, and pain in other body parts (e.g., neck, arm, or throat).

Recognizing and Reacting to Signs of a Heart Attack

Reducing the risk of a heart attack is the main goal of drawing aware-ness to coronary artery disease. However, if a heart attack should occur, what should someone do? What are the symptoms? How fast should you react and who should be contacted if you suspect you are having a heart attack?

The actions taken during the first minutes of a suspected heart attack are vital and could very well be the difference between life and death or long-term disability. Immediate emergency medical attention is warranted. Therefore, persons should know the early warning signs of a heart attack:

- Chest pain—often described as a squeezing or pressure that does not resolve with rest
- Pain that spreads to the shoulders, arms (especially left arm), and jaw
- Sudden shortness of breath
- Nausea, even vomiting
- Profuse sweating
- Lightheadedness

While chest pain is often the most recognized sign of a heart attack, such chest discomfort may be absent in certain populations, such as the elderly and women. Thus, it is important that people understand a heart attack may not always involve chest pain.

If these warning signs are experienced for more than a few minutes, the initial action should be notifying emergency medical services. Calling 911 is crucial; you should not attempt to drive or be driven by an individual who is not a paramedic. Ambulance transport to the hospital is important, as close monitoring, as well as medications, can be given during this time; lethal heart rhythms can be treated immediately; and patients with chest pain who arrive by ambulance receive faster treatment at the hospital.

Suggestions for Congregational Programs

Sponsor a program on heart disease. Invite a physician to speak about heart disease. Although a cardiologist may seem like an obvious choice, internists and family practitioners are well prepared to speak on the subject of heart disease. This may also be a good opportunity to offer blood pressure screenings as well as samples of low-fat and low-sodium foods.

Provide information on nutrition. A healthy diet is key to preventing and managing heart disease. Consider inviting a dietitian to speak on how to read a food label, and to offer advice on food selections and preparation. A series of cooking classes overseen by a dietitian is another option. These classes should emphasize foods that are heart healthy. Congregation members could even consider putting together a book on heart healthy recipes (see our website for suggestions: www.hopkinsmedicine.org/jhbmc/building-hcp).

Provide assistance for people who want to participate in a program of regularly scheduled physical activity. Distributing information on exercise programs available in the community is one way to draw attention to the importance of physical activity. Additionally, consider holding a scheduled physical activity at the congregation—a walking club, a hiking club, or yoga. The American Heart Association is a good resource for helping design exercise programs.

Offer a workshop or class on stress management. While stress itself was not highlighted earlier in this chapter as a risk factor for coronary artery disease, anxiety and stress are common and may be modifiable risk factors. So, organizing sessions on stress management focused on meditation, arts, or physical activity such as yoga could be considered.

Offer a class on cardiopulmonary resuscitation (CPR) and automated external defibrillators (AED). If a heart attack should occur, having members of the congregation who know CPR could save a life. The American Heart Association or the local hospital can arrange to provide a class on bystander CPR. Encourage all from the congregation to attend but especially those who are caregivers caring for older adults. Training could also include how to use AEDs, which are often present in large public facilities (e.g., airports, shopping malls, and sports arenas). Consider purchasing an AED and training several congregational members on how to use it in case of an emergency.

Provide information on smoking cessation. Smoking is one of the most important behaviors to change, and stopping smoking is among the most challenging human health problems Encourage congregation members who smoke to talk with their health provider about the best methods to stop smoking. Also, consider placing in a highly visible area of the congregation information about 1-800-QUIT NOW (1-800-784-8669), a nationwide program that provides a variety of resources for individuals interested in smoking cessation.

Provide information on recognizing and responding to signs of a heart attack. Consider distributing handouts, available from the American Heart Association, to the congregation.

Consider implementing Heart Health Fairs for the congregation and/or the community. This fair could include screenings, from blood pressure to cholesterol, as well as information on nutrition, cooking, and even CPR. Teaming up with the American Heart Association and/or a local hospital for such a fair is wise in order to provide adequate resources for the event.

Examples of Congregational Programs

Each February, St. Matthew United Methodist Church in Turner Station, Maryland, holds a "Red Dress Sunday." Congregation members are encouraged to wear red, the color designated by the American Heart Association for heart health, and they receive handouts with information about heart disease. One particularly meaningful Red Dress Sunday included a presentation by a physician, followed by a question-and-answer period. The pastor, Reverend Dred Scott, then made a promise in front of the congregation to talk to his health care provider to make sure he is doing enough for his own heart, and he asked others to do the same.

The congregation at St. Matthew was so motivated by what they had learned at another of their Red Dress Sundays that they organized a three-hour educational session on a Saturday afternoon focused on what persons can do to combat heart disease. Discussions covered weight loss, exercise, and diet. At the end of the sessions, they made a promise to lose weight before the next Red Dress Sunday. To help with this, they organized walks and shared recipes on heart healthy meals. After one year, the congregation had lost a total of more than 1,000 pounds, which was proudly illustrated on a poster in their lobby.

While preventing heart disease is crucial, it is important to recognize that people will still be diagnosed with this disease and may even suffer a heart attack. Therefore, it is vital for persons to know CPR, as this skill can save lives. At Mount Calvary AME Church Family Life Center in Baltimore, they are teaching their congregants how to implement bystander CPR. This initiative was driven by a few high school students, who believe that learning CPR is the equivalent of having a "super power."

Information Resources

You can obtain many of the resources discussed here from your local hospital or from your local American Heart Association chapter. To find the nearest chapter, visit the organization's website (www.americanheart.org) or call 1-800-AHA-USA-1 (1-800-242-8721). Both the organization and local hospital can help identify health professionals willing to present and lead CPR classes, as well as perform screenings.

Note that Red Dress Sunday for St. Matthew United Methodist Church took place in February, the month that the American Heart Association sponsors a national campaign to raise the public's awareness of heart disease. Consider scheduling a similar event in February to coincide with this education initiative.

Additional information on heart disease can be found at these websites:

www.cdc.gov/heartdisease (Centers for Disease Control and Prevention)
www.nhlbi.nih.gov/health/health-topics/topics/cad (National Heart, Lung, and Blood Institute)

For more information and resources, along with additional examples of congregational health programs, please visit the book's website at www
.hopkinsmedicine.org/jhbmc/building-hcp.

7

Hypertension

Hypertension, also known as high blood pressure, is a common condition in the twenty-first century. Blood pressure refers to the force of the blood against the walls of arteries. The more blood a heart is pumping into narrowed arteries, the higher the person's blood pressure will be. Blood pressure is also affected by the size and elasticity of the arteries. Two numbers are used to evaluate blood pressure—systolic and diastolic. **Systolic blood pressure** is the pressure when the heart is contracting, sending blood forward, and thus represents the higher blood pressure value. **Diastolic blood pressure** is the pressure when the heart is relaxed and filling with blood, and thus represents the lower blood pressure value. High blood pressure is generally defined as a systolic pressure of 130 mm Hg (millimeters of mercury) or higher or a diastolic pressure of 80 mm Hg or higher. Given the seriousness of hypertension, health professionals also encourage individuals to be aware of **elevated blood pressure**, a condition that often develops into hypertension if not given proper medical attention. Elevated blood pressure is defined as a systolic pressure of 120–129 mm Hg and a diastolic pressure of less than 80 mm Hg. Blood pressure categories are as follows:

- Normal: systolic pressure less than 120 mm Hg and diastolic pressure less than 80 mm Hg
- Elevated: systolic pressure 120–129 mm Hg and diastolic pressure less than 80 mm Hg
- Hypertension Stage 1: systolic pressure 130–139 mm Hg or diastolic pressure 80–89 mm Hg
- Hypertension Stage 2: systolic pressure 140 mm Hg or greater or diastolic pressure 90 mm Hg or greater

Hypertension affects nearly half of American adults, meaning more than 100 million adults have this serious condition. The likelihood of developing hypertension increases with age, with more than three-fourths of adults 65 years of age or older affected by it. Other risk factors for developing hypertension include race/ethnicity (African Americans have the greatest risk), a family history of hypertension, and overweight/obesity.[1]

The Risks of Ignoring Information on Hypertension

Although hypertension frequently produces no symptoms, it can have many serious health consequences, including severe disability and death.. During the asymptomatic or "silent" period, the high pressures are damaging both large and small arteries directly. This damage leads to disease in the tissues and organs receiving blood from the arteries. The damage can result in strokes, heart attacks, and kidney disease (which can lead to the need for **dialysis**). Hypertension also may lead to heart failure, as the heart muscle must work harder and can become overdeveloped and thickened, resulting in reduced pumping efficiency. People with heart failure from hypertension may tire easily and experience shortness of breath with even minor exertion.

Although hypertension frequently produces no symptoms, it can have many serious health consequences, including severe disability and death.

What Can Be Done to Prevent Hypertension and Its Complications?

Given the widespread occurrence of hypertension and the fact that it often produces no symptoms until it has seriously damaged the heart, brain, or kidneys, it is important that people be screened for the condition. Fortunately, the assessment of blood pressure is easy and inexpensive. In addition to having it checked at your health provider's office, you can check it yourself at automated monitors that are easy to use in many drugstores and grocery stores. Regular screening is especially important for those who have certain risk factors that cannot be changed—individuals with a family history of high blood pressure, older adults, and African Americans. Although these individuals are at greater risk of developing hypertension, they should not be discouraged. There are other risk factors—modifiable risk factors—that they can influence and thus reduce their chances of developing hypertension or at least allow them to control their condition and reduce the risk of complications. Modifiable risk factors associated with the development of hypertension include being overweight, not staying physically active, using tobacco, and consuming too much alcohol. Diet, especially one high in sodium (salt), also has been linked with hypertension development as well as impacting the ability to control the disease.

The good news about hypertension is that the interventions that can be used to prevent it also treat it. Once it is diagnosed, lifestyle modifications are frequently effective in controlling blood pressure. These include weight loss, restriction of salt intake, exercise, smoking cessation, and reduced alcohol consumption. These lifestyle modifications are generally recommended as an initial method of controlling blood pressure, but if such changes fail to bring blood pressure under control, numerous medications are available. If medication is needed, it is still recommended that individuals continue with their lifestyle modifications.

One of the greatest challenges in the treatment and control of hypertension is the difficulty many individuals have following their health care provider's recommendations. Studies have shown that only about half of the individuals with hypertension have it under control. There are many reasons for this problem, sometimes referred to as noncompliance or nonadherence. Because many people do not have any symptoms and the benefits of keeping their blood pressure under control are generally long-term, not immediate, they may feel little motivation to continue with the recommended lifestyle changes or medication. Also, some individuals stop or cut back on their medications because of unpleasant side effects, while others mistakenly believe that once their blood pressure has reached a healthy level they no longer need to stay on medication or continue with their lifestyle changes. And for some, the cost of the medication may be an obstacle.

Suggestions for Congregational Programs

Offer blood pressure screenings throughout the year, before or after congregational gatherings. Frequent monitoring of blood pressure assures that the individuals will be able to track their blood pressure more accurately. Further, it allows retired health care professionals (such as nurses) from the congregation to be able to continue using their skills in order to serve the community. Also, hospitals and home health agencies may be able to offer staff to conduct these checks or be willing to train volunteers to do so. In addition to screenings at the congregation, consider handing out or displaying information about where community members can obtain blood pressure checks (e.g., local drugstores, fire stations).

Sponsor a special program on hypertension with a physician or nurse educator as your featured speaker. Materials for such a program are available on our website (www.hopkinsmedicine.org/jhbmc/building-hcp), and additional materials can be obtained from the American Heart Association.

Use congregational bulletins, mailings, websites, and social media to provide members with basic information on hypertension. This information can be found on our website or obtained from the American Heart Association.

Use congregational bulletins, mailings, websites, and social media to provide members regular reminders about monitoring their blood pressure and complying with treatment recommendations.

Encourage people interested in controlling hypertension to participate in exercise or nutrition programs. Suggestions can be found in chapter 18 and on our website.

Examples of Congregational Programs

At St. Nicholas Greek Orthodox Church in Baltimore, a congregational health event was held on a Sunday after the worship service. This event followed a celebration of a national Greek holiday, thus guaranteeing a large audience. A major part of the event was blood pressure screenings offered by resident physicians from a nearby medical center. In order to set the tone and demonstrate the importance of monitoring one's health, the priest, Father Michael Pastrikos, volunteered to be the first person to have his blood pressure checked. Approximately half of the congregation followed his lead, with many also welcoming suggestions and advice about lifestyle changes that could help them control blood pressure.

Another example of a congregational program on hypertension was one held at St. Casimir Roman Catholic Church in Baltimore. The program was organized by a member of the church who had no formal education as a health professional but a strong interest in helping others stay healthy. To prepare for this congregational event, she participated in a training program on hypertension offered by nurses and physicians at a nearby hospital. In addition to being given a good overview of hypertension, she and other participants learned how to reliably measure blood pressures by using an automated monitor. They also received informational materials that she was able to distribute to members of the congregation.

Information Resources

The American Heart Association has local chapters throughout the United States. You can find the closest one through the organization's website (www.americanheart.org) or by calling 1-800-242-8721. Also, the American Heart Association or a local hospital may be able to identify professionals, volunteers, and other organizations able to assist with congregational or community educational programs and screenings.

Additional information on hypertension can be found at the following websites:

www.LowerYourHBP.org
www.cdc.gov/bloodpressure (Centers for Disease Control and Prevention: High Blood Pressure Fact Sheet)

For more information and resources, along with additional examples of congregational health programs, please visit the book's website at www .hopkinsmedicine.org/jhbmc/building-hcp.

8

Lung Disease

Lung diseases have a significant impact on the health of the US population. While there are many types of lung disease, the most common, and the focus of this chapter, are **asthma** and **chronic obstructive pulmonary disease (COPD)**. Both of these respiratory conditions can result in significant shortness of breath mainly caused by narrowing of the airways (the bronchi of the lungs) or, in the case of **emphysema** (a disease that can cause COPD), destruction of the **alveoli** (the sacs where oxygen is taken up by the blood). Asthma is an episodic problem, and during an attack, the muscles of the bronchi constrict, leading to narrowing of the airways. This narrowing can be so severe that shortness of breath occurs even at rest, impairing oxygenation and carbon dioxide clearance, which can be severe enough to cause death. In COPD, the smaller airways are usually narrowed because of excess inflammation and mucus production (as seen in **chronic bronchitis**, a disease that can cause COPD), and in addition, in some cases there is destruction of lung tissue (as seen in emphysema). So patients with COPD can be short of breath all of the time, while also experiencing exacerbations or flares related to episodic increases in small airway inflammation that can be brought on by infections or exposure to irritants.

Asthma affects people of all races and ethnicities, young and old alike. According to the Centers for Disease Control and Prevention, 1 in 12 adults and 1 in 11 children have asthma, and worldwide it is estimated that 300 million persons are affected.[1] Asthma is a condition where your airways become narrow and swell and often produce extra mucus. Such airway issues in asthma often lead to symptoms that include wheezing (an audible whistling heard near the chest coming from the lungs), coughing, and trouble breathing. While there is no known cure for asthma, most people can control their symptoms and lead normal lives. Control of asthma involves lifestyle changes as well as medications at times. Lifestyle changes include avoidance of triggers that patients recognize will lead to an asthma attack. These can include house dust, mold, animal dander or other environmental allergens, strong odors, smoking, weather changes, or even **gastroesophageal reflux disease (GERD)**. If avoidance alone does not improve symptoms, then patients may be prescribed inhalers and other medications.

Who Is at Risk?

Although asthma can occur at any age, childhood onset is typical, and the incidence in younger people is increasing. In particular, asthma rates among African American children grew 50 percent from 2001 to 2009. It is important for patients to discuss with their health care providers if they are having trouble breathing or frequent periods of coughing, which can be a sign of new-onset asthma, regardless of age. Asthma can be a stand-alone disease, but it also can be associated with other diseases, such as with allergies and allergic **rhinitis**. To determine if you have asthma, a detailed history of symptoms is the first step. Afterward, health care providers may order other tests (such as lung function tests, called **pulmonary function tests**) and have patients keep a record of their symptoms or test how much air they can blow out quickly (peak flow) in what is called a **peak-flow diary**.[2]

Those who are at greatest risk for developing COPD are current and former smokers. While there are other causes of COPD, tobacco use continues to be the primary cause of COPD in over 80–90 percent of cases. Usually a diagnosis of COPD is determined based upon the patient's history, but the severity of the disease is best assessed with lung function testing, often called pulmonary function tests.[3] Other diagnostic tests are also ordered and may include imaging of the chest with a chest X-ray and/or chest CT scan.

The Risks of Ignoring Information on Asthma and COPD

Millions of people who have COPD or asthma have ongoing symptoms that prevent them from performing their daily activities.[2, 3] Poorly controlled COPD and asthma can lead to days missed from work and school and even death. Patients with COPD or asthma are also at risk of having exacerbations, or a sudden worsening of their symptoms. Exacerbations are characterized by more coughing than usual and more difficulty breathing. These exacerbations can result in hospitalizations, and in some severe cases, death. However, exacerbations can be prevented with proper medical attention and one key step: stopping smoking. If diagnosed with asthma or COPD, discuss with your health care provider the best ways to prevent an exacerbation, and if you smoke, ask for strategies and resources to help you stop.

What Can Be Done to Prevent Asthma and COPD and Their Exacerbations?

In regard to asthma, there are no known ways to keep this disease from occurring. For COPD, as mentioned earlier, the major risk factor is smoking. Stopping smoking is key to preventing COPD from occurring, or if one has COPD, keeping it from worsening. Smoking can also make controlling asthma difficult and should be avoided by patients with asthma.

The importance of helping patients stop smoking and helping children avoid exposure to smoking cannot be emphasized enough. Parents who smoke around children with asthma put them at risk for troubled breathing, which may result in missed school days and even hospitalizations. Parents need to be educated about the hazards of smoking, and any misconceptions (e.g., smoking outside is safe as long as it is not around the child) must be corrected. People who have developed COPD because of their use of tobacco will need resources to help them stop smoking. Stopping smoking "cold turkey," for instance, may work for some but not others. Awareness initiatives, educational programs, and other resources focused on smoking cessation can make a significant impact on asthma and COPD. Suggestions and strategies for helping people stop smoking can be found in chapter 18.

The importance of helping patients stop smoking and helping children avoid exposure to smoking cannot be emphasized enough.

Vaccinations against infections known to target the lungs are another way to prevent exacerbations of asthma and COPD. Having a lung disease, even if there are no active symptoms, places individuals at higher risk for complications from the flu and pneumonia. Strategies focusing on flu and pneumonia vaccinations can help in preventing these infections from causing exacerbations in people with asthma or COPD. Discussions should be held with one's health care provider regarding the best time to receive these vaccines.

Other steps that may be helpful controlling asthma and COPD symptoms include modifications in a person's home and lifestyle. For example, indoor air pollutants have been found to be linked to poorly controlled asthma and COPD symptoms. In rural areas, cooking with wood and coal in homes with poor ventilation often produces high levels of particulate matter and nitrogen dioxide, which in turn lead to worsening asthma and COPD symptoms. Raising the awareness of the impact of home indoor pollutants can lead to proper action to help improve the air quality. In regard to lifestyle, obesity and diet have been shown to contribute to poor asthma and COPD control. Lifestyle changes should focus on good dietary habits and regular exercise. These lifestyle changes will have a beneficial impact on the body as a whole, not just the lungs.

Suggestions for Congregational Programs

Offer information and programs focused on reducing tobacco dependence. Stopping smoking can be extremely difficult for many people, even if they are experiencing ill effects from smoking and know they need to quit. Providing information about smoking cessation programs and resources, along with offering ongoing encouragement and support, can help them meet this challenge.

Organize vaccination programs. As the flu season approaches, provide information in bulletins and other congregational materials about the important role flu and pneumococcal vaccinations can play in preventing exacerbations. If possible, work with your public health department or a local pharmacy to offer vaccinations immediately before or after worship services.

Offer information about assessing and improving air quality in homes. It is important to increase awareness of the impact home air quality can have on respiratory diseases. This is especially true of secondhand smoke, which can worsen a person's asthma and COPD.

Offer exercise programs. Diet and weight have an impact on respiratory diseases, especially COPD and asthma. Exercise programs can help people achieve and maintain a healthy weight. Additionally, yoga has been shown to be beneficial to patients who have asthma or COPD because of its focus on breathing.

Examples of Congregational Programs

An "ask a doc" session focused on COPD and asthma was held at St. Paul Community Baptist Church in Baltimore during its annual "Thanksgiving in May" event, a program open to congregants and others living in the neighborhood. May is Asthma Awareness Month, so it was perfect timing to have a lung health conversation at the church. The "ask a doc" session was introduced by Reverend Dr. Gregory Perkins, who highlighted that a private room was reserved for participants to speak with the physician that day. Participants shared their concerns about their symptoms, especially how these conditions impact their daily lives. Further, fears of exacerbations were addressed, as one congregation member discussed how frightening it had been when a COPD exacerbation caused him to be on life support with a breathing machine for several days. The main skill taught that afternoon was how to properly use asthma and COPD medications, namely, handheld inhalers. Several participants, though reluctant at first, mentioned that they did not know how to use their inhaler, so a short instructional video about proper use of inhalers was shown. Finally, it was discussed that if patients continue to struggle using their medication, especially children using inhalers, then they should ask their health care provider for a spacer (a device that makes it easier for inhaler medication to reach the lungs). Pamphlets and handouts were distributed at the end of the presentation, with over 20 participants staying the entire time. Because of the success of the event, Dr. Perkins discussed a return of the "ask a doc" session in November (since it is COPD Awareness Month).

Another helpful program on lung health was a presentation on COPD held at the Mary Harvin Transformation Center at Southern Baptist Church in Baltimore. This session, led by a pulmonologist (lung doctor), focused on three key objectives: what the lungs do, how COPD impacts the lungs, and ways to improve breathing if you have COPD. The participants were able to see how the lungs work through a video, which was followed by another video showing how lungs are impacted by COPD. But most important, in the section on "ways to improve breathing," smoking was the main topic discussed. The members revealed their current smoking habits and struggles with smoking cessation. Several discussed past attempts at quitting cold turkey. Each participant agreed that quitting smoking is a hard thing to accomplish, but it could be easier if they tried to do it together. The lung doctor shared with them resources they could use to help quit smoking and promised to follow up in three months to see how they were doing. Pledge cards to quit smoking were handed out at the end in order to extend the enthusiasm about quitting smoking beyond the conclusion of the session.

Information Resources

Additional information on lung diseases can be found at the following websites:

www.chestnet.org/Foundation/Patient-Education-Resources/Asthma
(Chest Foundation Asthma Educational Resources)
www.chestnet.org/Foundation/Patient-Education-Resources/COPD (Chest Foundation COPD Educational Resources)
www.lung.org (American Lung Association)

For more information and resources, along with additional examples of congregational health programs, please visit the book's website at www.hopkinsmedicine.org/jhbmc/building-hcp.

9

Diabetes Mellitus

The number of Americans with diabetes mellitus, a condition defined by abnormally high levels of glucose (a natural sugar) in the blood, has grown dramatically in recent decades. In 1980, fewer than 6 million Americans were living with diagnosed diabetes.[1] By 2015, that number had climbed to more than 23 million, and each year there are almost 1.5 million new cases of diabetes diagnosed.[1] If this trend continues, by 2050 one out of every three adults in the United States will have diabetes.[1] Also alarming is the statistic that about 8 million people with diabetes do not know they have the disease.[2]

Diabetes impacts some groups more than others. For instance, 25 percent of adults age 65 or older have diabetes. The prevalence rates are even higher among Hispanic/Latino Americans and African Americans. Besides those diagnosed with diabetes, more than 85 million other Americans have **prediabetes**, or evidence of problems controlling glucose levels that increases their risk of developing diabetes and other serious problems, including heart disease and stroke.[1]

> About 8 million people with diabetes do not know they have the disease.

There are two major types of diabetes mellitus. **Type 1 diabetes**, also known as insulin dependent diabetes or juvenile diabetes, accounts for 5 percent of all diagnosed cases of diabetes in US adults. While type 1 diabetes can occur at any age, it is most likely to occur in persons under 20 years of age. There is no known way to prevent type 1 diabetes, as it is an **autoimmune disorder** in which the beta cells of the pancreas (the cells that create insulin) are destroyed. **Type 2 diabetes** is more common and is also known as adult-onset diabetes, as it is generally found in persons 40 years of age or older. Weight is a significant risk factor for type 2 diabetes, with overweight and obese adults at higher risk to develop this disorder. And with the current obesity epidemic in the United States occurring across all age groups, type 2 diabetes is becoming more common in children and adolescents, with more than 5,000 new cases of type 2 diabetes being diagnosed in persons 20 years old and younger every year. However, it should be noted that even lean adults can develop type 2 diabetes—usually associated with family inheritance. Other types of diabetes exist, such as gestational diabetes, which occurs during pregnancy; however, for this chapter we focus on type 1 and type 2 diabetes, as they are more common conditions.

In people with diabetes, **hyperglycemia** (high glucose levels) occurs because of a breakdown in the normal process of transferring glucose from a person's bloodstream into the body's cells and tissues. Insulin, a hormone produced by the pancreas (specifically, the beta cells of the pancreas), plays a critical role in the movement of glucose (sugar) from the blood into the cells. High levels of blood glucose result when the pancreas does not produce enough insulin (as is the case in type 1 diabetes) or when the cells are resistant or unresponsive to insulin (as is the case in type 2 diabetes).

Type 1 diabetes usually develops rapidly, with individuals experiencing unexplained weight loss, frequent urination, and excessive thirst over days, weeks, or months. Sometimes, type 1 diabetes, before it is diagnosed, can result in a potentially lethal condition known as **diabetic ketoacidosis** (also known as DKA). DKA often has symptoms of excessive nausea with or without vomiting, slow respirations, and confusion. DKA is a medical emergency, but upon presentation to the hospital it usually is rapidly diagnosed and successfully managed. Type 2 diabetes develops more gradually, often without any symptoms early in its course. Although individuals may experience few or no symptoms for several years, diabetes still can be damaging organs such as the heart and kidney during this time. Some symptoms that type 2 diabetes can cause include an increase in thirst and urination, visual disturbances, fungal rashes, and darkening of the skin around the back of the neck or in the armpits. While patients with type 2 diabetes also can develop diabetic ketoacidosis and another hyperglycemia emergency (hyperosmolar hyperglycemic syndrome), the more serious concerns of type 2 diabetes are associated with the long-term complications affecting other essential organs.

Who Is at Risk?

It is important that people at high risk for developing diabetes have the appropriate screening tests. At least two screening tests separated by a few days or weeks must be abnormal to make and confirm the diagnosis of diabetes. (Sometimes diet, medications, illnesses, or even anemia [low blood count] can cause abnormal test results in those who do not have diabetes, and thus having a second test is a necessary step in diagnosis.) There are three tests that can be performed to diagnose diabetes: a fasting glucose check, an oral glucose tolerance test, and a **hemoglobin A1c (HgbA1c)** test.[3] For the fasting glucose check, a patient is required to have had no food for at least 10 hours (often overnight) before blood is drawn and tested. Normal values for glucose are 100 mg/dL or less; a value of 126 mg/dL or more is diagnostic of diabetes. For an oral glucose tolerance test, the same procedure as for a fasting glucose test is initially followed. But in addition, after the first blood is drawn, the patient drinks a sugary mixture and has a second blood sample drawn two hours later. If the fasting blood glucose is 126 mg/dL or greater or if the blood glucose two hours later is 200 mg/dL or greater, a diagnosis of diabetes can be made. As for the final test, the HgbA1c gives an average level of blood glucose over the past two to three months. An HgbA1c less than 5.7 percent is considered normal; 6.5 percent or greater is considered diagnostic of diabetes.

Persons at risk for developing diabetes include adults over the age of 45, those with a family history of diabetes (type 2 diabetes has a strong genetic predisposition), certain races and ethnicities (Asian Americans, African Americans, Hispanics/Latinos, Native Americans, Pacific Islanders), persons who are overweight or obese, women with a history of gestational diabetes, and women with a diagnosis of polycystic ovarian disease.[1, 2, 3] Individuals who are at high risk for diabetes must advocate for themselves and ask their health care provider if it is appropriate to screen for diabetes.

The Risks of Ignoring Information on Diabetes

The millions of people who have diabetes but are not receiving treatment are at risk for many of the chronic complications of diabetes. Undetected and untreated diabetes sets the stage for other diseases or conditions that can kill or cripple:

- Stroke. Older adults with diabetes are almost twice as likely as those without diabetes to have a stroke.

- Heart disease. Older adults with diabetes are at least twice as likely to develop cardiovascular disease, and heart attacks in diabetes are more likely to be fatal.
- Eye disease. Cataracts, glaucoma, and retinopathy (damage to the retina) are more common among older adults with diabetes. Retinopathy can cause bleeding in the eye, leading to blindness.
- Kidney disease. Adults with diabetes are more likely to develop nephropathy (kidney damage) that often leads to kidney failure and the need for dialysis.
- Amputation. The risk of lower-extremity amputation is close to ten times greater for older adults with diabetes as compared to adults without diabetes.

The millions of people who have diabetes but are not receiving treatment are at risk for many of the chronic complications of diabetes.

What Can Be Done to Prevent Diabetes?

Currently there are no tests that can identify those at risk for type 1 diabetes, and there are no interventions that can prevent its development. Fortunately, the development of type 1 diabetes occurs with much less frequency than type 2 diabetes, and individuals at risk for type 2 diabetes are easy to identify. Since obesity and inactivity are the two most potent risk factors for developing type 2 diabetes, those who are overweight or obese and inactive should undergo regular screening tests to check their blood glucose levels. Such tests can help identify prediabetes, which should be viewed as an early warning sign and serve as motivation to make meaningful lifestyle changes to prevent the progression to diabetes. Individuals found to have prediabetes who then lose weight (even just 5–7 percent) and become more active are less likely to develop type 2 diabetes.[2] In fact, even among individuals who are overweight, regular exercise can improve glucose control, thereby likely postponing the development of diabetes, even without weight loss.

If either type 1 or type 2 diabetes is detected, some of the long-term complications can be eliminated, or postponed, or have their severity greatly reduced with treatment. Although treatment of type 1 diabetes includes daily injections of insulin, many cases of type 2 diabetes do not require insulin injections. If insulin is required, a patient may rely on insulin injections or even an insulin pump (a small, pager-like device worn on the waistband or belt that is programmed to deliver insulin through an attached catheter or thin plastic tube inserted under the skin). Type 2 diabetes often can be managed through a combination of diet, weight control, and exercise. Oral medications may be needed if diet and exercise do not adequately control the blood glucose levels. Some persons with type 2 diabetes will require insulin therapy to control the blood glucose levels. Insulin therapy should not be viewed as a punishment but as a valuable medication that can accomplish the important goal of returning the high blood glucose levels to near normal levels and preventing complications.

Although it may seem that people who are diagnosed with type 2 diabetes have a relatively simple treatment regimen to follow, many find it difficult to follow their health care provider's recommendations consistently. It is not easy to make major lifestyle changes, especially when there are no immediate, noticeable consequences. Changes in established patterns are difficult to make and even more difficult to maintain; therefore, patients need the ongoing encouragement and support of family, friends, their community, and their health care providers. Ultimately, achieving the best control over diabetes will have to involve attention to lifestyle (dieting and exercising) with or without medications (by mouth and/or insulin therapy). Well-controlled diabetes is a key part of avoiding the major complications of diabetes.

Suggestions for Congregational Programs

Sponsor glucose level testing. Work with representatives from a local hospital's medical laboratory or other community medical laboratories to arrange on-site testing. If this testing cannot be done at your facility, see if you can arrange for transportation to the hospital or medical laboratory.

Sponsor a special program on diabetes with a physician, nurse educator, or dietitian as your featured speaker. Provide snacks appropriate for persons with diabetes.

Offer support groups for patients and families affected by diabetes. Support groups can assist patients in following treatment recommendations and also in coping with some of the emotional challenges often associated with diabetes. Groups often are especially helpful for children diagnosed with type 1 diabetes. Additionally, in many communities there are summer camps and activities where they can meet other children facing the same challenges they are encountering. Your hospital or the local American Diabetes Association chapter can assist you in establishing a support group or in locating support groups in the community.

Sponsor or help members of your congregation locate exercise and weight-reduction programs. Most people find it easier to sustain their exercise or weight reduction efforts if they are part of a group.

Offer cooking classes for patients and families affected by diabetes. A hospital dietitian or the American Diabetes Association can assist with materials and other resources for this program.

Use congregational bulletins and mailings to provide members with basic information on diabetes. This information can be obtained from our website (www .hopkinsmedicine.org/jhbmc/building-hcp) or from the American Diabetes Association. Your local chapter and your local hospital can provide copies of brochures and booklets to distribute.

Use church bulletins and mailings to provide members with regular reminders about exercise, dieting, glucose monitoring, and complying with their medication regimens.

Examples of Congregational Programs

Sacred Heart of Jesus / Sagrado Corazón de Jesús Catholic parish in Baltimore is the spiritual home for a large and rapidly growing Latino population, a group that is known to have one of the highest rates of diabetes. Recognizing the need to address this serious health problem, the church's priest and lay leaders welcomed the opportunity to partner with physicians and other health professionals from Johns Hopkins Bayview Medical Center. One of the key programs that emerged from this partnership was an initiative titled Yo Puedo ("I Can"), where participants could learn about diabetes and the steps they could take to reduce their risk of developing diabetes or, if they already had been diagnosed with diabetes, to manage their condition effectively and thus reduce the risk of complications. To demonstrate the support of physicians and other health professionals and to reinforce the key message to members of the community that preventing and managing diabetes is in their control, the Yo Puedo project began with a kickoff event at the hospital. Several speakers, from primary care physicians to endocrinologists to dietitians, spoke on the importance of managing diabetes. Following the kickoff event, weekly sessions, all offered in Spanish, were held at the church. Participants learned about nutrition, exercise routines that could be done in their homes and neighborhoods, and strategies for weight management. At one session, families were invited to bring their favorite foods in order to find out how much sugar and calories were in these items.

Yo Puedo was enthusiastically embraced by the Latino community and led to the creation of an annual event called Mueveton, which is held at a local park. During Mueveton, a full day is dedicated to exercising and educational programs on proper dieting and nutrition.

Another example of a community-based program on diabetes was organized in collaboration with Southern Baptist Church in Baltimore, a largely African American congregation. Recognizing that African Americans, especially those over 65 years of age, have a high risk of developing diabetes, the program was held at the church's senior housing center. The discussion focused primarily on dietary ways to improve diabetes management. The guest speaker, a physician representing Medicine for the Greater Good, explained the importance of paying close attention to nutrition labels and understanding how much sugar should be consumed with each serving and within a day. Further, attention was drawn to the food label's "serving size," something that often is overlooked. Healthy foods, such as fruits and vegetables, were also discussed, along with an explanation of how sugars in these items impact glucose levels as compared to sugars found in processed foods. Dietary changes, such as choosing water over sugary soda products, were suggested, and participants were given a handout that provided further guidance on food labels and healthy food choices.

Information Resources

Your local chapter of the American Diabetes Association can provide much of the information and many of the materials you will need for your programs. You can locate the nearest office of the American Diabetes Association by visiting its website (www.diabetes.org) or calling 1-800-DIABETES (1-800-342-2383). The American Diabetes Association or your local hospital may be able to help identify professionals, volunteers, and other organizations in your community that offer services such as guest speakers for congregational and community programs, support groups for patients with diabetes and their families, educational classes, and information on medical supplies.

The American Diabetes Association sponsors a national diabetes awareness campaign every November. You may wish to schedule a congregational program on diabetes to coincide with this national campaign.

Additional information on diabetes can be found at the following web-sites:

www.cdc.gov/diabetes/data/ (Centers for Disease Control and Prevention—Diabetes Information)

www.niddk.nih.gov (National Institute of Diabetes and Digestive and Kidney Diseases)

For more information and resources, along with additional examples of congregational health programs, please visit the book's website at www.hopkinsmedicine.org/jhbmc/building-hcp.

10

Kidney Disease

The kidneys are best known for their ability to filter wastes and excess fluids from blood, which are then excreted in urine, but they also help regulate blood pressure, maintain electrolyte and mineral balance, produce a form of vitamin D, and even help the body produce red blood cells. A diagnosis of kidney disease (often called renal disease or renal failure) means that a person's kidneys are damaged, resulting in their inability to filter blood effectively. **Chronic kidney disease** or **chronic renal failure** (often referred to by the initials CKD or CRF) develops over many years and can lead to end-stage kidney disease, resulting in the need for dialysis or a kidney transplant. Chronic kidney disease affects approximately one of every seven Americans, with higher rates found among African Americans and Hispanic/Latino Americans.[1, 2] The rates of chronic kidney disease are also higher among women than among men. (Although kidney damage can occur rapidly and result in acute kidney or renal failure from drug toxicity, rare infections, or other unusual autoimmune disorders, rapid-onset kidney failure will not be covered in this chapter.)

> Chronic kidney disease affects approximately one of every seven Americans, with higher rates found among African Americans and Hispanic/Latino Americans.

Kidney function is usually first assessed by blood work. During this assessment, a physician will evaluate two blood products that the kidney filters from the blood: blood urea nitrogen and creatinine. These markers provide important information about the function of the kidneys. If they are abnormally high, a workup will begin that will attempt to answer why kidney function has changed, and to see if this change can be treated. Additional tests for kidney disease include collection of a urine sample to check for loss of proteins and also may include imaging of the kidneys (for example, by ultrasound).

The two most common causes of chronic kidney disease are diabetes and high blood pressure. Having a family member with kidney disease can also raise a person's chances of developing it. The encouraging news is that with proper control of one's blood sugar and blood pressure, kidney disease can often be prevented or the impact of kidney disease can be minimized. Other causes of kidney damage include overuse of certain medications, conditions such as lupus and HIV, and even an enlarged prostate, which can block normal urine flow in men. If your physician determines that you have kidney disease, a thorough investigation for possible reversible causes will begin.

Chronic kidney disease is staged from 1 through 5. Sometimes in the earlier stages (1–3), action can be taken to prevent kidney disease from getting worse. Unfortunately, less than 10 percent of those who have early stage chronic kidney disease are aware of their condition.[1] This is because of the fact that the early stages of kidney disease often have few, if any, symptoms. Thus, without proper screening at routine check-ins with one's health care provider (with blood and urine tests), kidney disease in its early stages may be missed. At the advanced stages (stages 4 and 5), patients must begin considering initiating dialysis or being assessed for a kidney transplant, as there is often no therapy to reverse the damage.

The Risks of Ignoring Information on Kidney Disease

As mentioned, one of the risks of ignoring kidney disease is missing the opportunity to reverse it and/or stop its progression. Without stopping kidney disease's progression, you may end up needing a kidney transplant and/or dialysis. Close to 500,000 Americans are on dialysis, and 200,000 Americans are living with a functioning kidney transplant.[2] Chronic kidney disease also increases the chance of a stroke or heart attack. Further, kidney disease can lead to death, as kidney disease now kills more people in the United States than either prostate cancer or breast cancer. Therefore, ignoring information about the prevention, diagnosis, and treatment of kidney disease can result in significant mortality and **morbidity**.

What Can Be Done to Prevent Kidney Disease and Its Complications?

First, knowing your risk of kidney disease is important. The two main risk factors are diabetes and high blood pressure (also known as hypertension); however, two additional risk factors are family history of kidney disease (an indirect way of learning about one's genetic makeup) and cardiovascular disease (such as a prior heart attack or stroke).[2] These four risk factors increase one's chances of developing kidney disease. Other risk factors for developing kidney disease include race and ethnicity (African Americans, Hispanics/Latinos, and Native Americans are at an increased risk of kidney disease), age (people over the age of 60 are at increased risk), obesity, and certain diseases, such as lupus and sickle cell anemia. Therefore, knowing your risk can help you assess what the appropriate action for screening and lifestyle changes will include.

Being aware of the subtle symptoms of early kidney disease is also important. Although most people with chronic kidney disease do not have any severe symptoms until their disease has reached an advanced stage, there are a number of signs and symptoms of kidney disease that may be noticed and that should prompt a discussion with your health care provider. The National Kidney Foundation lists the following possible signs and symptoms:

- Feel more tired and have less energy
- Have trouble concentrating
- Have a poor appetite
- Have trouble sleeping
- Have muscle cramping at night
- Have swollen feet and ankles
- Have puffiness around your eyes, especially in the morning
- Have dry, itchy skin
- Need to urinate more often, especially at night

It should be noted that these symptoms are nonspecific to kidney disease, meaning they could be caused by other diseases. Nevertheless, if you have some of these symptoms, discussing them with your health care provider is important in order to determine if they are being caused by kidney disease or other diseases.

There are certain risk factors, such as age and family history, that a person cannot control. However, there are several steps people can take to prevent or better manage their kidney disease and preserve their kidney function. These include monitoring blood pressure and blood sugar levels, avoiding or limiting medications that are known to injure kidneys (e.g., some over-the-counter painkillers), and preventing infections when possible (such as through annual flu vaccinations), as infections can result in kidney damage. Other healthy actions include exercising, maintaining a healthy weight, eating a diet rich in fruits and vegetables, following up regularly with a health care clinician, monitoring and controlling cholesterol levels, and quitting smoking.

There are several steps people can take to prevent or better manage their kidney disease and preserve their kidney function.

Suggestions for Congregational Programs

Organize presentations on kidney disease and kidney health. February is often highlighted as Heart Awareness Month, and congregations plan many activities during this month to recognize heart disease. March is Kidney Month, and similar events can be conducted to raise awareness of kidney disease, especially in African American and Hispanic/Latino congregations. Inviting a kidney specialist, called a nephrologist, to talk about kidney health and how to prevent kidney disease is a good way to promote awareness about this often silent disease.

During programs on kidney health, perform blood pressure screenings. Just as blood pressure screenings at programs on heart disease can help people understand the connection between high blood pressure and heart disease, blood pressure screenings at programs on kidney health can help people see the link between high blood pressure and chronic kidney disease.

Use congregational bulletins and mailings to provide members with information on kidney disease and screenings and what they can do to improve kidney health. Materials can be obtained from the National Kidney Foundation or your local hospital. Consider March to distribute the material, as this month is the designated National Kidney Month.

Organize or help people locate support groups for people who are on dialysis or have had kidney transplants. Undergoing dialysis or having a kidney transplant can be taxing on an individual and on family members, and support groups can provide people with encouragement and helpful resources.

Examples of Congregational Programs

Southern Baptist Church in Baltimore, a largely African American congregation, and the National Kidney Foundation of Maryland worked together to offer a special program on kidney disease—Kidneys: Evaluate Yours (KEY). This program, provided at no cost to the church or individual participants, was held after the Sunday worship service in the church's fellowship hall. More than 80 members of the congregation, including the church's pastor, Reverend Dr. Donté Hickman, took advantage of the program, where participants first met with a nurse to be weighed, have their blood pressure taken, and review their family and medical history. They then were seen by a phlebotomist, who drew a blood sample that would be sent to the medical laboratory. The results of the blood work were mailed to each participant approximately two weeks later. The results were also sent to the medical director for the National Kidney Foundation of Maryland, a nephrologist, who contacted those individuals whose results indicated their kidneys were not functioning normally. The medical director discussed their results in detail and provided guidance about the steps they should take to determine why their kidney function had changed and to see if the change could be treated.

At Sacred Heart of Jesus / Sagrado Corazón de Jesús Catholic Church in Baltimore, local physicians and the church's spiritual leaders decided to make a special effort during the month of March (National Kidney Month) to share information about kidney health and kidney disease with Hispanic/Latino members of the congregation and community, a group known to be at higher risk for developing kidney disease. This outreach effort included inserts in the church bulletin, pamphlets distributed to businesses and organizations in the community, an article published in the local Spanish language newspaper, and screenings. The screenings included blood pressure evaluations, weight assessments, and family history discussions. All materials and presentations were offered in Spanish. Also, advice on cost-effective health access was provided in order to allow people to seek more extensive screenings for kidney disease. At the first event of the month-long initiative in 2014, over 30 Hispanic/Latino family members attended a presentation on kidney disease and had their blood pressures checked. At the end of the presentation, participants were given an opportunity to make a pledge to discuss with their health care provider if they were at risk of developing kidney disease and when kidney disease screening would be appropriate. Follow-up programs on kidney disease continue to be held at Sacred Heart of Jesus / Sagrado Corazón de Jesús, with the information being offered in English and Spanish.

Information Resources

The National Kidney Foundation is a valuable resource for information on kidney disease, with materials offered in English and Spanish. Information can be found on its website (www.kidney.org) or obtained by calling toll free 1-855-653-2273.

Additional information on kidney disease can be found at these websites:

www.niddk.nih.gov (National Institute of Diabetes and Digestive and
    Kidney Diseases)
www.cdc.gov/diabetes/programs/initiatives/kidney.html (Centers for Disease Control and Prevention: Chronic Kidney Disease)

For more information and resources, along with additional examples of congregational health programs, please visit the book's website at www
.hopkinsmedicine.org/jhbmc/building-hcp.

11

Cancer

There are more than 100 types of cancer, all characterized by the uncontrolled growth and spread of abnormal cells that have the potential to invade and destroy normal body tissue. At first, most solid cancers are localized, with cancer cells confined to their original site. However, over time, these cancer cells may spread, or **metastasize**, to other parts of the body. Some less common cancers of the bloodstream, such as leukemia, involve the body more generally at the time of presentation. The most common cancer types that lead to death include lung, breast, colorectal, and prostate. Skin cancers are by far the most common type of cancer, especially among older adults, but less frequently lead to death. Treatments for cancer can be most effective when the cancer is localized; once cancer has spread, treatment is more difficult and less effective.

The prevalence of cancer is likely to increase in the next few decades because of two factors: an aging population (cancer rates increase with age) and an increasing obesity epidemic (cancer rates increase with weight). Therefore, encouraging discussions on cancer prevention and early diagnosis through screenings can save lives.

More than 1.6 million new cases of cancer are diagnosed in the United States each year, and close to 600,000 Americans die from cancer annually. Deaths from cancer have decreased over the last 20 years (by 1.8 percent among men and 1.4 percent among women) but still remain higher for African Americans than for non-Hispanic/Latino whites, reflecting differences in genetics, environmental exposure related to socioeconomic status, and health care disparities.[1] Paralleling these differences, the five-year survival rate for cancer in African Americans is significantly lower than for non-Hispanic/Latino whites, due in large part to diagnosis occurring later in the disease process.

The Risks of Ignoring Information on Cancer

The fear of being diagnosed with cancer is common. This fear often prevents people from obtaining accurate information about cancer and the appropriate ways to prevent it. Many individuals are so fearful of cancer that they do not want to know much about it or participate in screenings that might detect it. Often, this fear is combined with a fatalistic view of cancer—a belief that there is little that can be done to prevent cancer and that there are virtually no effective treatments. People need help in overcoming their fear and sense of hopelessness about cancer. In recent years, screening for cancer has become more precise, and early detection has reduced some cancer death rates. The main risk of ignoring the risk of cancer and avoiding cancer screenings is that a potentially treatable and manageable cancer disease is not discovered until it progresses to an advanced stage, where treatment may be far less effective. People need to know that there are steps they can take to reduce the risk of developing cancer, especially advanced cancer, and that these steps can result in cures.

What Can Be Done to Prevent Cancer?

It is important that cancer be detected and treated as early as possible. Generally, the earlier the treatment begins, the better the chance of curing or controlling the cancer. The overall survival rate for many cancers would increase significantly if more people participated in early detection programs. A combination of regular self-exams and screenings provides the best means of detecting cancer early enough to allow for effective treatment. Unfortunately, too many people ignore or are not aware of the recommendations about regular self-exams and screenings.

> **It is important that cancer be detected and treated as early as possible.**

Currently, there are several cancers that have available screenings. The American Cancer Society[2] recommends the following screening tests:

- Breast cancer screening: This is accomplished by mammograms. Currently, it is recommended that women of average risk between the ages of 40 and 44 discuss the risks and benefits of screening with their primary care physician. Women with a parent, sibling, or child with breast cancer are at higher risk for breast cancer and thus may benefit more than average-risk women from beginning screening in their forties. All women between the ages of 45 and 54 are recommended to undergo screening with mammograms every year. At age 55, women may consider mammogram screenings every other year or continue with their annual screening. These screenings should continue as long as a woman is in good health and can expect to live 10 or more years.

■ Colon and rectal cancer screening: Starting at the age of 50, both men and women should undergo a colorectal screening test. The gold standard is a colonoscopy, as it evaluates the entire colon and rectum, and may offer the ability to remove precancerous lesions; however, colonoscopies carry risks with them that are associated with anesthesia and the procedure itself. Less invasive tests include a flexible sigmoidoscopy; however, this test does not evaluate the entire colon and may miss cancer lesions at other parts of the colon. Finally, radiographic tests for colorectal cancers (double-contrast barium enema tests or CT colonographies) could be used for screening. The issue here is that if a polyp is seen, a colonoscopy will be recommended for further evaluation. Colonoscopy screenings, if negative, can be done every 10 years, while the other studies should be performed every 5 years. There are also tests that can look just at one's stools (a fecal occult blood test or stool DNA testing). Individuals should discuss the various tests with their health care provider to see if they are an appropriate candidate for them.

■ Cervical cancer screening: Women, beginning at the age of 21, should have cervical exams, called Pap tests, every three years. Beginning at the age of 30, women can have Pap tests every five years with concurrent screening for human papillomavirus (HPV). After the age of 65, women who have had regular cervical cancer testing in the past 10 years with normal results may consider stopping the test. Note that even if one has received a vaccine against HPV, the common virus known to cause cervical cancer, women still should undergo these cervical cancer screening tests.

■ Lung cancer screening: This screening test, essentially a CT scan of the chest, is only recommended for high-risk patients. A high-risk patient is someone aged 55 to 74 who has a long smoking history (the equivalent of one pack per day for 30 years) and is either still smoking or has quit within 15 years.

- Prostate cancer screening: Starting at age 50, men should talk with their health care provider about the benefits and risks of prostate cancer screening. While there are tests—a PSA (prostate-specific antigen) blood test and a rectal exam—for prostate cancer screening, current research is undecided if the benefits of these tests outweigh the risks associated with testing and treatment. Therefore, it is recommended that men discuss their family history and any current symptoms with their health care provider before deciding whether or not to be tested.

- Testicular cancer screening: Testicular cancer is more common in young men, and it is recommended that screening be done from age 16 or around the onset of puberty to age 40. Men should discuss with their health care provider the appropriate way to perform self examinations and report to their provider any worrisome findings. Physical examination by a health care provider is the gold standard in screening, and if there are abnormal findings, further imaging tests can be performed.

- Skin cancer screening: While this is not recommended for everyone, persons with a strong family history of skin cancer, especially melanoma, and/or significant sun exposure should discuss with their health care provider if they should have a skin exam.

For each of these screening recommendations, high-risk patients (e.g., strong family history) should discuss with their health care provider if they should begin screening earlier than the recommended age.

Some people fail to participate in regular screenings for cancer because of their fear of the pain or indignities associated with screenings. Therefore, accurate information about the nature of the screenings and the definite benefits of early detection need to be provided. Special efforts are needed to increase the number of African Americans and Hispanic/Latino Americans who participate in early detection programs. Historically, lower rates of participation among minority groups have resulted in later detection of cancers and higher mortality rates than among non-Hispanic/Latino whites. Efforts should be focused on assuring that all persons receive the appropriate screenings, with more attention on specific populations who do not take advantage of these life-saving interventions.

The American Cancer Society[2] has developed the mnemonic CAUTION to help individuals recognize potential warning signs of cancer:

C: Change in bowel or bladder habits

A: A sore that does not heal

U: Unusual bleeding or discharge (such as vaginal bleeding or blood in one's urine)

T: Thickening or lump in breast or other regions of one's body

I: Indigestion or difficulty swallowing

O: Obvious change in an old wart or mole

N: Nagging cough or hoarseness in one's voice

Note that the CAUTION symptoms are not specific for cancer, as they can be caused by other problems. Therefore, it is important to discuss these issues with one's health care provider, especially if these symptoms persist beyond two weeks.

People also need to be aware that their risk of developing cancer may be reduced by making modifications in their lifestyle—most importantly, stopping smoking. The American Cancer Society estimates that more than 80 percent of lung cancer deaths result from smoking, and that almost 175,000 cancer deaths each year can be attributed to the use of tobacco. However, even longtime smokers who quit have a reduced risk (compared with people who continue smoking) of lung, laryngeal, esophageal, oral, pancreatic, bladder, and cervical cancer. Excessive alcohol consumption also can increase the risk of cancer. It has been associated with esophageal, stomach, and liver cancers. Finally, there are occupational exposures that may put persons at risk for certain cancers. Individuals should discuss with their health care provider if they are concerned that their work environment poses any risk for cancer development.

Diet can play an important role in reducing the incidence of cancer. Diets high in fat or low in fiber may play a causative role in cancer, whereas the daily consumption of vegetables and fruits is associated with a lower risk of lung, prostate, bladder, esophageal, and stomach cancers.

More than half of the cases of colon cancer, a disease that affects both men and women, occur after 70 years of age.

Many people do not realize that the chance of getting cancer increases with age. For example, breast cancer is thought by many to be a disease that primarily affects middle-aged women. In fact, the incidence of breast cancer rises steadily with age, and more than half of women who develop breast cancer do so after 65 years of age. Therefore, it is important for older women to have regular physical examinations and mammograms. Similarly, more than half of the cases of colon cancer, a disease that affects both men and women, occur after 70 years of age.

How Can Cancer Be Treated?

Many people believe that there are no effective treatments for most types of cancer or that the available treatments are worse than the disease. Consequently, it is important that they be given honest, accurate information about treatments and their right to choose treatments. Patients should be encouraged to ask their health care providers about treatment options, including their risks and side effects, as well as the expected benefits of the treatments and the likely consequences of no treatment. The approaches to cancer treatment are increasingly complex and require the expertise of oncologists, or even oncology specialists (physicians who gain expertise in caring for a limited number of cancer types). Treatment modalities are diverse, continuously evolving, and can include infusion of intravenous medications (usually called **chemotherapy**), oral drugs, radiation therapy, hormonal suppression therapy, and biologic agents engineered to treat a specific cancer. The newest approaches using genetic "fingerprints" to guide treatment for some tumors and "immunotherapy" for other types such as lung cancer hold particular promise. The side effects of treatment also require attention, and multidisciplinary cancer programs should have expertise in ensuring that these adverse consequences are anticipated, minimized, and promptly addressed.

Support groups can be helpful to those with cancer and to their families and friends. They can provide valuable emotional support, and there is evidence that cancer patients who participate in support groups live longer.

Suggestions for Congregational Programs

Offer educational initiatives focused on available screening tests. This initiative should focus on types of screening tests available, appropriate ages for screening, and an emphasis on gathering one's family history. While handing out materials is important, having members from the congregation discuss their experience being screened can be very powerful and allay some fears and concerns.

Provide help for congregation members who wish to stop smoking. A support group is a great way to encourage current smokers to stop smoking. Emphasize 1-800-QUIT NOW for more resources. Congratulating ex-smokers in the congregation also may help reinforce the importance of taking on this challenge.

Take advantage of cancer awareness months. Choose Hope (www.choose hope.com) has a list of which months are set aside for specific cancers in order to raise awareness. For example, October is Breast Cancer Awareness Month, November is Lung Cancer Awareness Month, and September is Prostate Cancer Awareness Month. Congregations can take advantage of these months to educate their congregations on how to be screened for these cancers and how to prevent them (e.g., a smoking cessation campaign in November).

Provide skin cancer screenings. Use these screenings as an opportunity to encourage people to talk with their health care provider about other screenings they should pursue.

Sponsor a presentation on cancer. An oncologist or medical professional who is regularly involved in the diagnosis or treatment of cancer can serve as your featured speaker. The American Cancer Society can provide materials to distribute at this program.

Sponsor support groups for people affected by cancer. Congregations can look into offering support groups for persons who have been affected by cancer. Potential leaders for support groups include hospital social workers, mental health professionals, nurses, and cancer survivors. If a congregation is unable to hold its own support group, sharing information about local support groups is another way to help community members.

Examples of Congregational Programs

One example of a cancer screening conversation occurred at St. Nicholas Greek Orthodox Church in Baltimore. There, a primary care physician discussed that if one wanted to be "cured from cancer," then screening for cancer should be a priority for everyone. The program was presented in both English and in Greek in order to be understood by all congregation members. The priest challenged everyone in the audience to pursue screening and invited the physician to return a year later. One year later, a woman from the congregation told her story of her first colonoscopy, performed two months after the prior year's cancer talk, and how three polyps were found and removed. She began crying in front of the audience because she felt that her life had been saved by this early intervention. This powerful story has resulted in the congregation requesting annual talks on cancer screenings.

St. Matthew United Methodist Church in Turner Station, a largely African American community near Baltimore, sponsored an event featuring an oncologic nurse practitioner who presented on breast cancer. She spoke to this audience in order to highlight how many lives could be saved if more African American women sought mammograms as recommended. Instead, African American women often are not diagnosed and do not receive treatment until they have advanced breast cancer. The nurse practitioner finished her passionate talk with handouts describing how women can schedule a mammogram test.

Information Resources

The American Cancer Society (www.cancer.org) can provide material for the aforementioned suggestions. To find a local chapter, call 1-800-ACS-2345 (1-800-227-2345).

The American Cancer Society or your local hospital can also assist in identifying professionals, volunteers, and other organizations in the community that can provide additional resources for community programs and/or support groups.

Additional information and materials on cancer can be found at these websites:

www.cancer.gov (National Cancer Institute)
www.cdc.gov/cancer (Centers for Disease Control and Prevention)

For more information and resources, along with additional examples of congregational health programs, please visit the book's website at www.hopkinsmedicine.org/jhbmc/building-hcp.

12

Depression

Clinical depression (also referred to as major depression or major depressive disorder) is a serious condition that affects millions of Americans every year. It is significantly different from the periods of sadness or feelings of grief that occur as an expected part of life for most people. Although it is normal to be sad or "down" occasionally and to experience grief when a significant loss occurs, clinical depression has more severe symptoms, often lasting for a long period of time, and is more likely to have an impact on a person's ability to function normally.

It is estimated that during any given month almost 5 percent of Americans will experience an episode of major depression, and the lifetime prevalence is more than 17 percent.[1] When other depressive conditions such as bipolar disorder and persistent depressive disorder are included, the estimate of lifetime prevalence exceeds 20 percent.[1] In other words, one of every five Americans will experience at least one serious episode of depression at some point in his or her life. Females are generally thought to be about twice as likely as males to experience major depression, but no group is exempt from this painful illness. Depression can be found among the young and the old, the religious and the nonreligious, and all ethnic and racial groups.

> One of every five Americans will experience at least one serious episode of depression at some point in his or her life.

Depression is not only painful but can also greatly impair a person's relationships and ability to work productively. In many cases, it is a life-threatening condition, placing people at risk for death from suicide or physical conditions such as heart disease.

One of the most unfortunate and tragic aspects of depression is that, in spite of the availability of several effective methods of treatment, it frequently goes undetected and untreated. Often the symptoms are incorrectly thought to be caused by medical conditions or other factors—particularly aging. Even when people are aware of their depression, they may underestimate the seriousness of the disorder or feel hopeless about ever finding effective treatment.

Because depression is so frequently undetected, it is important for congregational health education programs to inform their members about the symptoms of depression. The most common symptoms are:

- Depressed mood with overwhelming feelings of sadness and grief; and/or irritable mood
- Loss of interest and pleasure in activities formerly enjoyed
- Noticeable changes in appetite and weight (significant weight loss or gain)
- Insomnia, early morning waking, or oversleeping
- Restlessness or being physically slowed down
- Decreased energy or fatigue
- Feelings of worthlessness, guilt, or hopelessness
- Difficulty concentrating or thinking, indecisiveness
- Recurrent thoughts of death or suicide

A formal diagnosis of major depression is given when a person has experienced five or more of these symptoms every day or almost every day during a two-week period, and at least one of the symptoms is depressed or irritable mood or loss of interest or pleasure in activities previously enjoyed. This means that individuals could have a normal mood but still be clinically depressed if they have a loss of interest in formerly pleasurable activities and enough of the other symptoms.

Another form of depression is persistent depressive disorder. This is a milder but chronic pattern of depression. People with this disorder experience symptoms of depression for most of the day, more days than not, for at least two years. A third mood disorder in which a person experiences episodes of depression is bipolar disorder (also known as manic-depressive disorder). In addition to depression, the person experiences periods of mania or hypomania. The manic episodes are characterized by periods of abnormally and persistently elevated or irritable mood, along with excessive activity.

These episodes are severe enough to cause significant problems at work and at home. Hypomanic episodes involve milder manic symptoms. More information about both of these mood disorders is available on our website (www .hopkinsmedicine.org/jhbmc/building-hcp).

The Risks of Ignoring Information on Depression

The most serious consequence of failing to recognize and treat depression is the greatly increased risk of suicide. The tremendous emotional pain of depression, combined with the sense of hopelessness about ever obtaining relief from the pain, leads many people to see death as their only escape. Confused thinking, cognitive distortions, and concentration problems also contribute to suicidal thoughts and actions. Stated simply, people are not thinking clearly when they are depressed. Each year in the United States there are more than 40,000 suicides—more than twice the number of homicides—and the suicide rate has been increasing.[2] A recent analysis found that between 1999 and 2014 the suicide rate in the United States increased by 24 percent.[2] It was the second leading cause of death in the 15- to 34-year-old age group (after unintentional injury) and the fourth leading cause of death in those 35 to 54 years of age, but the group at greatest risk of suicide is older men.

Depression also can have a harmful impact on a person's physical health. For example, someone who has a heart attack and is depressed is more likely to die than the person who has a heart attack but is not depressed. It has also been found that people who are depressed have a greater risk of developing and dying from heart disease. This connection between depression and heart disease is likely due, at least in part, to the fact that depressed individuals, feeling hopeless and helpless about their situation, are less likely to take good care of themselves. In addition, depressed people are less likely to follow the treatment recommendations for other chronic conditions such as diabetes.

There is also the impact depression can have on family members. It often contributes to family conflict, difficulties at work, and financial problems. Too frequently we hear accounts of destructive or deadly actions that were caused, at least in part, by depression.

Recognizing and Responding to Depression

There are a number of obstacles that can interfere with depressed individuals getting the treatment they need. A common obstacle is that people do not recognize depression when they experience it or see it in others. Depression often goes undetected because we attribute some of the symptoms to other factors. For example, we may not be surprised when someone seems moody and withdraws from family and friends. We may assume that they just need some "time for themselves." Depression can be especially difficult to detect among the elderly. Older adults are less likely to report that they are depressed, and often their symptoms of depression are attributed to physical disorders or are thought to be a normal part of aging. Because of these difficulties in detecting depression, a congregational health program needs to find creative ways to share information so that people can recognize the symptoms of depression in themselves and others.

Although detecting depression can be difficult in any setting, religious congregations often offer opportunities to recognize and respond to it—if people know what to look for. Since one of the most common symptoms of depression is the inability to enjoy activities that previously brought pleasure, depressed individuals often stop attending worship services and other congregational activities. For example, they might drop out of the choir or stop attending a religious education class or a congregational social activity in which they have been regularly involved. In most cases, depression is probably not the reason for a change in their level of participation, but it could be why some individuals are no longer as active. This is when a call or visit in which someone from the congregation sensitively inquires about the person's change in congregational activities could help determine if he or she is depressed. If the individual explains that travel or other competing activities have interfered with congregational activities, then there likely is little reason to be concerned about depression. But if the person talks about a loss of interest or pleasure in these activities, then some follow-up questions about other symptoms of depression (e.g., sleep disturbance, decreased energy, changes in appetite) could help determine if the issue might be depression. If it is, then it is important to offer support and to encourage the individual to discuss what they are experiencing with their health care provider or a mental health professional.

But even when people do recognize depression, they do not always seek treatment. One reason is the stigma that many people still feel is attached to depression or any mental disorder. They believe that it is a sign of personal weakness or moral failure. Many believe that if only they were a better person or their faith were stronger they would not be depressed. Because of these beliefs, they are embarrassed to let others know they are depressed and to seek professional care. These beliefs can constitute a serious and dangerous barrier to treatment. A congregational health education program must find ways to eliminate or overcome this barrier.

Another obstacle that can stand in the way of treatment, even for those who recognize their depression and do not feel embarrassed about their condition, is the extreme pessimism and confused thinking that sometimes accompanies depression. It is not unusual for depressed individuals to feel hopeless about their situation, believing there is nothing that can be done to improve their lives. It is important that they be given hope by providing them with reliable, up-to-date information about treatment options and, when possible, examples of individuals who have been successfully treated for their depression. They need to learn about both biological and psychological methods. There are many effective medications available, but it is important for individuals to understand that antidepressant medications take time to work—at least two to three weeks to begin to work, with significant improvement often within six weeks. While most of these medications can be prescribed by a primary care provider, treatment by a psychiatrist may be appropriate and necessary when symptoms are severe or if there is a poor response to the medication initially prescribed.

There are also effective psychotherapies. Most of these therapies that have been demonstrated to be effective in the treatment of depression (e.g., cognitive behavioral therapy and interpersonal therapy) are relatively short-term and problem-focused. They do not involve years of treatment or a detailed examination of childhood issues. In fact, psychotherapy should produce noticeable improvement within six weeks. Psychological treatment in combination with antidepressant medication is especially effective in relieving depression.

Unfortunately, it is not unusual for individuals who have recognized that they are depressed and that they need professional care to then encounter another obstacle—difficulty getting an appointment with a mental health professional. Even individuals with good health insurance can find it challenging to locate a psychiatrist, psychologist, or other mental health professional who participates in their health insurance plan, and those without health insurance may find their options even more limited. Difficulty finding a provider can be frustrating and discouraging to anyone seeking the services of a health care professional but especially to a depressed individual who has little or no energy and is already feeling pessimistic about almost everything. This is where a family member, friend, or congregational volunteer can help by offering to assist in the search for mental health services.

Finally, in addition to removing the obstacles that often interfere with depressed persons receiving the treatment they need, a congregational program on depression should provide guidance and support for individuals who have loved ones who are depressed. It can be especially challenging to try to care for persons who no longer find pleasure in any of the activities they previously enjoyed and who are thoroughly pessimistic about ever feeling better. The National Institute of Mental Health (NIMH) offers the following suggestions for families and friends:

- The most important thing you can do is to help your friend or relative get a diagnosis and treatment. You may need to make an appointment and go with him or her to see the doctor.
- Encourage your loved one to stay in treatment or to seek different treatment options if no improvement occurs after six to eight weeks.
- Offer emotional support, understanding, patience, and encouragement.
- Talk to him or her, and listen carefully.
- Never dismiss feelings, but point out realities and offer hope.
- Never ignore comments about suicide, and report them to your loved one's therapist or doctor.
- Invite your loved one out for walks, outings, and other activities. Keep trying if he or she declines, but don't push him or her to take on too much too soon.
- Provide assistance in getting to doctors' appointments.
- Remind your loved one that with time and treatment, the depression will lift.
- Caring for someone with depression is not easy. Someone with depression may need constant support for a long period of time. Make sure you leave time for yourself and your own needs. If you feel you need additional support, there are support groups for caregivers too.

Suggestions for Congregational Programs

Raise your congregation's awareness of depression by placing information on the symptoms, prevalence, and treatment of depression in congregational bulle-

tins and mailings. Special attention should be given to the encouraging news about effective treatments for depression. Materials on these topics can be obtained from the National Institute of Mental Health, Mental Health America, the Depression and Bipolar Support Alliance, and the National Alliance on Mental Illness (NAMI).

Work toward reducing the stigma attached to depression by having respected leaders of your congregation emphasize that depression is a common disorder that does not reflect weakness or moral failure. It should be recognized and treated as a medical condition, not as a character flaw. The personal testimony of an individual who has experienced depression and knows the definite benefits of medical and psychological treatments can be especially effective.

Incorporate information on depression into regularly scheduled programs and activities. Many of the people who need information on depression may be reluctant to attend a special program on the subject. They may feel more comfortable if this information is provided in regularly scheduled programs.

Find opportunities for discussions on suicide among the various age groups in your congregation. People need to learn that the hopelessness felt by depressed persons often leads to suicide.

Publish in congregational bulletins and mailings the telephone numbers of the National Suicide Prevention Lifeline (1-800-273-8255—available 24/7) and other agencies where a person in distress can call or visit if he or she needs immediate assistance.

Examples of Congregational Programs

I (WDH) am frequently invited by congregations to give a presentation on depression, a topic that has interested me since graduate school and that has taken on special significance in my life since it has had such a devastating impact on my family (see at the end of this chapter the op-ed I published in the *Baltimore Sun*). Although for most of my presentations I have spoken from the perspective of a clinical psychologist who has been involved in the diagnosis and treatment of depression, there have been occasions when I have felt it was appropriate to also talk about what it was like when I became seriously depressed in my late thirties and then again in my midfifties. One of the reasons I have at times shared my personal experiences is to help remove or at least diminish the stigma that is still too often attached to depression. The other reason I have talked about my depressive episodes is to help people understand how painful and debilitating the experience can be and how hopeless everything can seem but also how there are effective treatments for depression and how the support of family and friends is important when one is in the dark depths of a depression.

A few weeks after one of my presentations at which I had discussed my own experiences, I received a note from a woman who had attended my talk. She wrote that her attendance at this program marked the first time she had been in her church for several months. She had stayed away, she said, because she felt utterly worthless and that there was nothing in her life for which she felt thankful and nothing to look forward to. It would feel "wrong" for her to be in her church, where others seemed so full of joy and hope, and she was certain other people would not want to be around her. But when she read in the church newsletter that there would be a program on depression, she decided to make the effort to attend. She went on to say that it was during my presentation that she first began to see at least a little ray of hope about her situation. If someone else had felt as bad as she did and then gone on to recover and return to an active, fulfilling life, perhaps she could, too. And the encouraging information about the benefits of antidepressant medication and psychotherapy gave her further hope.

Armed with the information about treatments for depression, she had made an appointment with her family physician, who agreed that she was depressed and prescribed medication. Her physician had also referred her to a psychologist known for her work with depressed individuals. She concluded by saying that with the help of the medication and her therapist, she had begun to emerge from her depression and was on her way back to being the sociable and confident person she had been before sinking into her depression.

Another informative congregational program on depression took place one Friday evening following the Shabbat service at Temple Beth El in Ormond Beach, Florida. At the end of the service, Rabbi Barry Altman introduced Dr. Maximo Handel, a psychiatrist and member of the congregation, who spoke for about fifteen minutes on many important aspects of depression. He described the symptoms, causal factors, and some of the treatments that are available. He pointed out that depression is a treatable condition but that often persons suffering from depression feel so hopeless and helpless that they fail to realize there are effective treatments available. He also pointed out that family members frequently fail to detect the signs of depression or attribute them to other causes. Dr. Handel emphasized the great importance of recognizing and treating depression because of the extreme pain and suffering it causes the affected individual, the detrimental impact it can have on relationships and work, and the increased risk of suicide. At the conclusion of the presentation, Rabbi Altman invited those who had questions to speak with Dr. Handel at the Oneg that would follow, and several members of the congregation used this opportunity to speak with him about personal concerns.

Information Resources

Your local affiliate of the National Alliance on Mental Illness (www .nami.org) or Mental Health America (www.mentalhealthamerica.net) can provide many of the materials you can use in your programs as well as information about other resources in your community (e.g., screenings and referrals, guest speakers for community programs, support groups for depressed persons and their families, support groups for persons going through various stressful experiences). Information and materials appropriate for use in congregational programs also can be obtained from the National Institute of Mental Health (www.nimh.nih.gov/index.shtml). A particularly informative booklet available on the NIMH website is *Depression: What You Need to Know*. This publication is in the public domain and may be reproduced or copied without permission from NIMH (www.nimh.nih.gov/health/publications /depression-what-you-need-to-know/index.shtml).

For more information and resources, along with additional examples of congregational health programs, please visit the book's website at www .hopkinsmedicine.org/jhbmc/building-hcp.

NOTE: The following op-ed appeared in the June 13, 2016 edition of the *Baltimore Sun*.

Three years ago I stood in the pulpit of the church where my family had worshipped for more than three decades to give the most difficult talk I have ever had to give—offering reflections on the life and death of my 36-year-old daughter, Libby, who had passed away just a few days before. As I prepared my remarks, Libby's sister and brother encouraged me to speak openly about the illness responsible for her death. If she had died of cancer, they noted, we would not be reluctant at all to talk about her battles with and eventual death from it. But it was not cancer that took Libby from us. It was another terrible disease—depression.

Depression was not unfamiliar to me. I am a clinical psychologist and have devoted much of my research and clinical work to mood disorders. And I have had personal experience with depression as well, having had two serious episodes that required medical and psychological treatment.

As I looked out over the more than 300 people attending the memorial service that evening, I didn't know what type of response to expect to my remarks about Libby's struggles with depression and how she had eventually taken her own life. But I felt strongly that I owed it to Libby and to all those still suffering from depression. It was time to use this dark moment in my life to shed light on this crippling and often lethal illness.

I must confess that I was surprised by just how many people spoke to my children and me after the service to express appreciation for my remarks—their words spoken with sincerity and purpose. The refrain, "we need to talk about depression," was repeated over and over again in these conversations. "We need to talk about depression in our schools." "We need to talk about depression in the workplace." "We need to talk about depression in our houses of worship." "We need to talk about depression in our homes."

I was truly heartened by these comments, and especially moved over the next few weeks when I learned that many of these concerned individuals followed up their words with donations to support the production of an educational video on depression that we chose to title, "We Need to Talk: A Story of Loss and Hope."

Since Libby's death, I have had many occasions to share this video and to speak about depression in educational institutions, religious congregations, and workplaces. I have used these opportunities to encourage audiences to view depression as an illness, just as they would diabetes or hypertension, and to recognize that there are effective treatments. I have focused particularly on two of the major obstacles that often interfere with depressed individuals seeking treatment: the stigma still too often associated with depression and the sense of hopelessness that is a central component of depression.

As I have given these talks, I have watched closely and listened carefully to discern the information or examples that have the greatest impact on my audiences. There is usually some interest in the research and clinical reports I provide, but it is clear that the most impactful part of my presentations is when I share my own experience with depression. There is something very powerful about having a professional speak openly, without any sense of shame or embarrassment, about his own struggles with depression and how, with treatment, he has been able to return to a full, active life.

As gratifying as it is when I see that I have helped people by talking openly about my depression, I must confess that I know I have passed up other opportunities where it would have been entirely appropriate and potentially quite beneficial for me to share my own experience. And I have had no reason not to. I know that I can speak candidly in these situations without jeopardizing my career or my most important relationships because my colleagues are fully aware of my mental health history, as are my wife, children, and closest friends.

While it is true that not everyone who has had a similar experience with depression can talk about it without concern for their employment or relationships, undoubtedly there are individuals from various walks of life—health care, education, religion, government and the business community—who, like me, have been successfully treated for depression and who could speak openly without fear of harmful repercussions. Imagine the impact we could have if more of those suffering in silence with the pain and despair of depression could hear our stories of how we were able to emerge from the dark, lifeless depths of depression and discover that our lives could once again include feelings of love, joy and hope.

What a powerful force we could be.

W. Daniel Hale

13

Dementia

Dementia is a clinical syndrome or condition in which there is a progressive deterioration of mental faculties, usually over many years. Problems with memory are typically the first sign of dementia. Other symptoms may include difficulties with language, impaired judgment, problems in performing simple tasks such as dressing, and changes in personality and behavior. It is common for people with dementia also to develop clinical depression, agitation, anxiety, or other behavioral symptoms as their disease progresses.

It is important for people to understand that dementia is not an inevitable consequence of aging. Although the risk of developing dementia increases with age, the overwhelming majority of older adults do not have dementia. Most older adults who report problems with memory do not have and may never develop dementia. Minor memory problems may be a normal part of aging and should not be seen as evidence of dementia.

> **It is important for people to understand that dementia is not an inevitable consequence of aging.**

There are a number of brain disorders that can result in dementia. The most common is Alzheimer's disease, accounting for 60–80 percent of dementia cases.[1] Alzheimer's is a progressive and degenerative disease that damages brain cells, especially in the regions responsible for memory and intellectual functions. Currently there is no cure for this progressive disease, although there are drug and nondrug treatments that can help with cognitive and behavioral symptoms.

Vascular dementia is the second most common cause of dementia, accounting for about 10 percent of dementia cases.[1, 2] The impact of vascular dementia on brain cells is caused by blood vessel issues. When these vessels are narrowed or blocked, there is a resulting lack of nutrients and oxygen going to brain cells, leading to small, damaged areas of the brain. Vascular dementia can be thought of as a compilation of many "small strokes" in the brain, resulting from blocked small arteries over a period of months to years. Vascular dementia and Alzheimer's disease often coexist and share some common modifiable risk factors, including hypertension, hyperlipidemia, obesity, diabetes, and smoking.

There are several potentially reversible conditions that can mirror symptoms of dementia. These include vitamin deficiencies (e.g., B12 vitamin deficiency), hormone abnormalities (e.g., **hypothyroidism**), and overmedication or unusual drug reactions.[1, 2] Additionally, depression is a common condition in the elderly, and its symptoms can be similar to dementia. Older adults who are depressed often have problems with their memory and social interactions and can experience moments of confusion. Distinguishing between depression and dementia is crucial, as they have different treatments, and with depression, appropriate treatment can actually reverse memory and social symptoms.

The Risks of Ignoring Information on Dementia

The potential harm of relying on inaccurate or incomplete information about dementia and the health care resources appropriate for managing this condition goes beyond the patient. Dementia is often referred to as a "caregiver's disease" because of its impact on family and friends. A person with dementia will need a loved one or loved ones to help with the many new challenges and stresses that, at times, may seem overwhelming and endless. Conflicts may arise within the family while caring for their loved one because of decisions and pressures that come with the disease, especially as it progresses. Also, it is not uncommon for family members to experience depression in reaction to this difficult situation. Family members who confront these challenges without the appropriate knowledge, skills, and resources are in danger of developing their own health problems.

The belief that dementia is inevitable and that there are no effective treatments for any type of dementia can have painful consequences for patients and their families. One potential consequence is that a person exhibiting symptoms commonly seen in dementia may miss the opportunity to have an alternative, and often reversible, condition diagnosed and treated. Additionally, many people believe that nothing can be done to prevent the development of dementia. Although there is no sure way to prevent the development of dementia, there are steps people can take that may reduce their risk and that are unquestionably good for their overall health, especially their heart. These include appropriate attention to the prevention or control of chronic conditions, such as diabetes and high blood pressure, along with regular exercise and proper nutrition. Stated simply, what is good for your heart is good for your brain, too.

Although there is no cure for dementia, there is still much that can be done to help patients and caregivers. Physical exercise and social activity are important in the management of dementia, as are proper nutrition, maintenance of overall health, and a calm and well-structured environment. For some of the most troubling symptoms of dementia, including depression, sleep disturbance, agitation, **delusions**, and **hallucinations**, there are medications and nondrug interventions (e.g., daily structure, behavioral management) that are helpful. Additionally, supportive care for people with dementia ensures that they are safe (e.g., through stopping driving, increasing supervision, preventing wandering); that they have a structured daily life plan; and that they are active. It also is important to provide supportive care for caregivers, making sure they are taught caregiving skills; that they are well educated about dementia; and that they have adequate respite.

What Can Be Done to Reduce the Impact of Dementia?

Although there is no cure for most of those diagnosed with dementia, there are ways to soften its impact on patients and their families. Many families initially wish to keep a loved one with dementia at home, but they soon become overwhelmed by the problems this condition presents. Families can overcome many of these problems if they have a good understanding of dementia and know some effective strategies. Fortunately, materials and programs are available that can provide families with information about how to better manage the home care of individuals with dementia. And there is encouraging research showing that families who learn about dementia and effective management and coping strategies often are able to delay placing their loved one in a nursing home, in some cases up to a year longer, compared to those without similar knowledge and resources.

Many families that are determined to keep their loved one at home become overwhelmed because they fail to use the services of various agencies and organizations in the community that offer assistance to people with dementia and their families. Respite care and adult day care programs can provide caregivers with much-needed relief from the seemingly constant demands of monitoring and caring for a cognitively impaired person. Unfortunately, families often are unaware of the many services and resources that are available.

Support groups are an important part of the care of people with dementia and their families. Many of the emotional conflicts and burdens associated with the constant care of a person with dementia can be eased by sharing feelings and information with others who face the same challenges.

Suggestions for Congregational Programs

Sponsor a special program on dementia. A neurologist, psychiatrist, psychologist, or other health care professional familiar with dementia can provide helpful information and should be able to respond to the various questions and concerns of the audience. You may wish to provide free blood pressure checks before or after the presentation on dementia. This will help people make the connection that hypertension can cause some forms of dementia.

Sponsor a special program on the community resources available to patients and families affected by dementia. This could include information about the various living arrangements appropriate for dementia patients at different stages of their condition. A social worker or case manager from a hospital, nursing home, or home health agency could serve as your featured speaker.

Compile a list of agencies and organizations in the community that offer services for individuals and families affected by dementia. This should include support groups, respite care programs, adult day care centers, and home health agencies.

Compile a list of books and materials that offer families advice on living with and helping loved ones with dementia. One book that should be on this list is *The 36-Hour Day: A Family Guide to Caring for People with Alzheimer's Disease, Other Dementias, and Memory Loss in Later Life* (sixth ed.) by Nancy L. Mace and Peter V. Rabins. Other helpful books can be found on our website (www .hopkinsmedicine.org/jhbmc/building-hcp).

Sponsor a support group for families with dementia. Consider offering a monthly support group that focuses on families affected by dementia. The support group can be facilitated by a mental health professional who has experience working with patients and families affected by dementia.

Sponsor a weekly or monthly "Caregivers Night Out" program. Families that are caring for a loved one with dementia often have few opportunities to meet their own social needs. Even if they are using adult day care, family members usually have to spend their evenings caring for and monitoring their cognitively impaired relative. Most would welcome the opportunity to have an evening to go out if they knew that their afflicted relative was receiving good care arranged by their congregation. Other suggestions for providing support for family caregivers can be found in chapter 21 and on our website.

Examples of Congregational Programs

A good example of a congregational program on the topic of caring for individuals with Alzheimer's disease is one coordinated by lay health educators representing four churches in the greater Daytona Beach area— Grace Episcopal, All Saints Lutheran, Westminster By-The-Sea Presbyterian, and Daytona Beach Christian and Missionary Alliance. The representatives organized an afternoon program on short- and long-term care options for individuals who have dementia or are physically frail. They put together a panel that included a physician who specialized in geriatrics, a discharge planner from a local hospital (Halifax Health Medical Center), the director of an adult day care center, and an administrator from an agency that provided in-home medical and personal care services. Dr. Jeffrey Sumner, the pastor of Westminster By-The-Sea Presbyterian Church, served as the moderator.

The geriatrician began the program and touched on many important aspects of medical care for cognitively impaired and physically frail persons. He also explained how factors other than the underlying illness must be considered when searching for long-term care options. For example, the functional abilities (ability to care for oneself) and the availability of a caregiver must be taken into account. The discharge planner then discussed the options she has when helping the patient and family identify the appropriate setting. Next, the director of the adult day care center described the services provided in that type of setting. She also handed out and reviewed a list of terms frequently used by professionals discussing care options for people with chronic illness. Finally, the administrator of the home health agency shared information on the medical and personal care services his organization could provide.

Dr. Sumner served as the moderator for the question-and-answer part of the program. The questions from the audience revealed that there was great interest in the topic and that many people were unaware of the resources in their community. It was clear that the lay health educators had provided a valuable service by bringing together a group of professionals whose expertise spanned virtually the entire range of issues on the topic of caring for cognitively impaired and physically frail elderly persons.

Another good example of a congregational program is the one held at the Masjid Al Ihsan in Baltimore, where Imam Hassan Amin organized a conversation about mental health and dementia for his community. This conversation, held after a Friday prayer service, was led by two physicians who spoke to the congregation about how the diagnosis of dementia is made and what family members can expect when a loved one is found to have this condition. They also provided information about health professionals and organizations that specialize in dementia care. It was evident that there was considerable interest in this topic, with many questions being asked and the speakers being invited to return for further discussion on dementia and related topics.

Information Resources

Many communities have a chapter of the Alzheimer's Association. You can call the national office of the Alzheimer's Association (1-800-272-3900) or visit its website (www.alz.org) to find the location of the nearest chapter. The Alzheimer's Association also provides a wide variety of materials and information about other community resources, including telephone help lines, support groups, and living arrangement options for people with Alzheimer's.

Another source of information and materials about Alzheimer's disease is the Alzheimer's Disease Education and Referral Center (www.nia.nih.gov /alzheimers, 1-800-438-4380), a service of the National Institute on Aging.

For more information and resources, along with additional examples of congregational health programs, please visit the book's website at www .hopkinsmedicine.org/jhbmc/building-hcp.

Child and Adolescent
Health Issues

The well-being of children and adolescents is important for every community, and religious congregations, working closely with health professionals and medical institutions, can provide much of the information and many of the resources parents and their children need. Here, we present several topics—obesity, mental health issues, substance abuse, and injuries—that impact the health and well-being of children and adolescents, and we offer suggestions for how medical-religious partnerships can address many of these important issues.

Childhood Obesity

Childhood obesity has increased dramatically in recent decades. Currently, almost 20 percent of school-aged children are obese, with the highest rates found among Hispanic/Latino and African American children.[1] This is a disturbing development because obesity places children at higher risk for a number of health conditions, including asthma and type 2 diabetes. Children with obesity also are more likely to have low self-esteem, experience depression and anxiety, and be bullied. Additionally, child obesity all too often leads to adult obesity, which carries with it the heightened risk of a number of serious medical conditions, including hypertension, heart disease, stroke, type 2 diabetes, and both breast and colon cancer.

> Obesity places children at higher risk for a number of health conditions, including asthma and type 2 diabetes.

Two major factors contributing to obesity are unhealthy eating patterns and physical inactivity. To address the first of these, children need to have access to nutritious foods and to understand that high-calorie foods and beverages (e.g., candy, desserts, sugar-sweetened drinks), if consumed in excess, can result in unhealthy weight gain. Learning to distinguish healthy from unhealthy foods is an important skill for children to acquire, as is learning what constitutes healthy portion sizes. But knowledge doesn't always lead to a change in habits, especially when it involves cutting back on favorite foods. For this reason, children need encouragement and support when they are trying to improve their eating patterns. Suggestions for working with children around the issue of healthy eating can be found on the Eat Right website (www.eatright.org) sponsored by the Academy of Nutrition and Dietetics and also on the Healthy Children website sponsored by the American Academy of Pediatrics, offered in English (www.healthychildren.org/english/pages/default.aspx) and Spanish (www.healthychildren.org/spanish/paginas/default.aspx).

Addressing the lack of exercise, the other major factor contributing to childhood obesity, is also important. Children who do not engage in regular physical activity (60 minutes every day is recommended by the Centers for Disease Control and Prevention) usually do not burn enough calories to maintain a healthy weight. Therefore, helping children become more active is an important way to prevent excess weight gain. Just as it can be difficult for children to change their eating habits, it can be challenging for children to give up some of their sedentary activities (e.g., television, video games). A number of excellent suggestions for how to encourage greater physical activity can be found on the Healthy Children website mentioned above.

Children do not exist in isolation but rather are dependent on their families for access to adequate, healthy food and for opportunities to exercise. For example, it is unrealistic to expect children to stop drinking soda while it's still available at home and being consumed by their siblings or parents. To help an obese child achieve a healthier weight, the entire household is likely to need to change their diet and exercise habits. Finally, concerns about the future health risks associated with obesity may not be meaningful to children. For that reason, focusing family and community conversations on the immediate benefits of healthy habits may be more relevant and lend a note of optimism to otherwise discouraging or difficult conversations.

Suggestions for Congregational Programs

Offer educational programs on healthy foods and beverages. Helping children distinguish healthy foods from unhealthy ones is a skill that can last them well into adulthood. Learning how to read the "nutrition facts" labels for most packaged foods and beverages is an important part of this. Including parents in these programs is important, as they are often making the decisions about what food to purchase for the home. Dietitians from local hospitals can be excellent resources for such programs and can provide suggestions for healthy snacks that can be part of the program.

Explore options for increasing access to healthy foods. If access to healthy foods is limited in the surrounding neighborhood or where many congregants live, your congregation can assist by working with food banks or grocers to have congregational facilities serve as a site where healthy foods can be purchased after worship services or other congregational gatherings. Also, explore connecting with local nonprofits to help eligible congregants connect with SNAP (Supplemental Nutrition Assistance Program) benefits.

Coordinate fun exercise events for children. Consider hosting weekly exercise sessions appropriate for the whole family that families could replicate on their own at home during the week. Also, during the summer months when children are away from school, sponsor regular fun events involving physical activity. Holding events centered on exercise is one way to offset a sedentary lifestyle that children may fall into when they do not have a structured school day.

Mental Health

Mental health issues often arise early in life and can present significant challenges for the affected children, parents, and others involved in their care. We first briefly review **autism spectrum disorder (ASD)** and **attention deficit / hyperactivity disorder (ADHD)**, both of which are familiar to pediatricians, teachers, and many parents. We then devote greater attention to depression and anxiety, two serious conditions that too often go unrecognized and untreated.

Autism spectrum disorder refers to a group of developmental disorders characterized by (1) difficulty communicating and interacting with others and (2) repetitive behaviors as well as limited interests and activities. Autistic disorder and Asperger's syndrome are no longer separate diagnostic categories, and individuals who previously were diagnosed with either of these disorders are now given the diagnosis of autism spectrum disorder. The symptoms of ASD may appear as early as infancy. The severity of the symptoms and the degree of disability can vary widely. Diagnosis relies on a medical examination and careful review of the child's history. Treatment for ASD often involves a variety of interventions, including behavior and communication therapies, structured educational programs, and family therapies. Medications may help with certain symptoms. Additional information about the symptoms, diagnosis, and treatment of ASD can be found on the National Institute of Mental Health website (www.nimh.nih.gov/health /topics/autism-spectrum-disorders-asd/index.shtml).

Attention-deficit / hyperactivity disorder is a condition that affects millions of children. Symptoms include difficulty maintaining attention, hyperactivity, and impulsive behavior. Symptoms can be mild to severe and may differ between boys and girls, with boys more likely to be hyperactive and girls more likely to be quietly inattentive. Symptoms of ADHD in a child may be predominantly inattention or predominantly hyperactive-impulsive behavior or a mixture of the two. Diagnosing ADHD relies on a comprehensive examination and detailed data gathering conducted by a pediatrician, psychologist, or other health professional with expertise in ADHD. Treatment for ADHD includes education, counseling, training, and, at times, medications. More information on the symptoms, diagnosis, and treatment of ADHD is available on the National Institute of Mental Health website (www .nimh.nih.gov/health/topics/attention-deficit-hyperactivity-disorder-adhd/ index.shtml).

One of the most serious mental health issues for adolescents is depression. While it is not uncommon for adolescents to feel sad at times, and perhaps use "depression" to describe how they are feeling, approximately 5 percent of adolescents will experience a much more serious emotional disturbance, a condition that health professionals refer to as either major or clinical depression. This is a medical illness that can lead to significant problems at home and school and that increases the risk of both substance abuse and suicide, the second leading cause of death among individuals ages 15 to 24. One of the greatest challenges about addressing the needs of adolescents who are depressed is that it often goes unrecognized and untreated. Even when it is recognized, many adolescents do not talk about what they are experiencing because they fear being criticized or judged by others. They also may be reluctant to seek the help of health professionals because they do not realize that there are effective treatments.

Congregations can play an important role by sharing information on the signs and symptoms of depression. The following list is provided by the Centers for Disease Control and Prevention:

- Feeling sad, hopeless, or irritable a lot of the time
- Not wanting to do or enjoy fun things
- Changes in eating patterns—eating a lot more or a lot less than usual
- Changes in sleep patterns—sleeping a lot more or a lot less than normal
- Changes in energy—being tired and sluggish or tense and restless a lot of the time
- Having a hard time paying attention
- Feeling worthless, useless, or guilty
- Self-injury and self-destructive behaviors

Along with providing information about the signs and symptoms of depression, it is important to emphasize that depression should be viewed as a medical illness, in the same way that asthma and diabetes are seen as medical illnesses, and not the result of personal failure or lack of willpower. Additionally, the message that this is a treatable illness needs to be conveyed. The treatments for adolescents who are depressed are the same as those for adults who suffer from depression. Information about these treatments can be found in chapter 12.

An excellent resource on this subject is the Adolescent Depression Awareness Program offered by the Johns Hopkins University Department of Psychiatry and Behavioral Sciences. Information about this program, including a helpful booklet, *Adolescent Depression: What We Know, What We Look For, and What We Do*, is available on the department's website (www.hopkinsmedicine.org/psychiatry/specialty_areas/moods/ADAP/).

Another important mental health issue for children and adolescents is anxiety. Although it is not unusual for children and adolescents to feel anxious about school or friendships or when they are facing new, unfamiliar situations, when these feelings of anxiety persist for weeks or months and interfere with their schoolwork or relationships with family and peers, this may be an indication that they have an anxiety disorder. It is estimated that about one in seven young persons will experience an anxiety disorder, but as with depression, anxiety disorders often go unrecognized and untreated.

Following are examples of anxiety disorders given by the Centers for Disease Control and Prevention:

- Being very afraid when away from parents (separation anxiety)
- Having extreme fear about a specific thing or situation, such as dogs, insects, or going to the doctor (phobias)
- Being very afraid of school and other places where there are people (social anxiety)
- Being very worried about the future and about bad things happening (general anxiety)
- Having repeated episodes of sudden, unexpected, intense fear that come with symptoms like heart pounding, having trouble breathing, or feeling dizzy, shaky, or sweaty (panic disorder)

These anxiety disorders can be extremely debilitating, but the good news is that there are effective treatments. More information on anxiety disorders and their treatment can be found on the website of the Anxiety and Depression Association of America (https://www.adaa.org/living-with-anxiety/children/childhood-anxiety-disorders).

What Can Be Done to Address These Issues?

Autism spectrum disorder, attention-deficit / hyperactivity disorder, clinical depression, and anxiety disorders are important health issues that religious congregations can help address. Left unrecognized, these mental health conditions can have a far-reaching impact on the affected individuals, as they often struggle academically and socially. Thus, it is important for congregations to talk openly about mental health issues, just as they would speak about any other health issues, and to provide reliable information about how to recognize each of these conditions and where to turn for a confirming diagnosis, treatment, and support.

Suggestions for Congregational Programs

Use bulletin inserts or articles in newsletters to provide information on each of these conditions. Information about these mental health issues can help families recognize what may be the early signs of the condition and then seek appropriate professional care. If there are health education programs at your congregation, include depression and anxiety as topics. Including depression and anxiety along with asthma or diabetes helps underscore the relevance of mental health to overall well-being.

Invite a mental health professional to speak about child and adolescent mental health issues. Consider holding this event on or close to National Children's Mental Health Awareness Day sponsored by the Substance Abuse and Mental Health Services Administration (SAMHSA) each year in the month of May. Information about this is available on the SAMHSA website (https://www .samhsa.gov/). Your local chapter of NAMI (National Alliance on Mental Illness) may be able to provide a speaker and materials for the program.

Offer or provide information on support groups for families with children and adolescents with ASD, ADHD, depression, or anxiety. Families with children who have ASD, ADHD, depression, or anxiety disorders often face serious challenges coping with these disorders. Sharing experiences with others in similar situations and learning about additional resources and coping strategies can be very helpful.

Substance Use Disorders

Adolescence is a time when the brain is vulnerable to substance use disorders. The National Institute on Drug Abuse (NIDA) has a helpful analogy, stating, "The adolescent brain is often likened to a car with a fully functioning gas pedal (the reward system) but weak brakes (the prefrontal cortex)."[2] And we know that the use of alcohol, tobacco, and illegal and prescription drugs by teenagers is not uncommon. The Youth Risk Behavior Survey, conducted by the Centers for Disease Control and Prevention and given to public and private high school students in the United States every two years, provides a good overview of the scope of the problem.[3] Because all of the questions are answered anonymously, this survey is considered a reliable way to determine rates of adolescent substance use. In 2015, 63 percent of high school students reported having tried at least one drink of alcohol, and 33 percent were currently drinking alcohol at the time of the survey. Thirty-two percent of students had tried a cigarette, although only 11 percent were smoking at the time of the survey. Thirty-nine percent of students had tried marijuana, and 22 percent of students admitted to smoking marijuana at the time of the survey. The opioid issue is also impacting adolescents as well, with 7.8 percent of high school seniors reporting nonmedical opioid use. It also has been found that only 1 in 12 adolescents and young adults who need care for any type of addiction receive treatment. These are troubling numbers and illustrate why this is such an important issue to address within our communities.

What Can Be Done to Address This Issue?

There is no one intervention to prevent or stop substance use in adolescence, but good communication and positive social support are key parts of most strategies. It is especially helpful to have family-centered discussions about substance abuse start in childhood. Because many parents find this difficult to do, group settings are often preferable. These group settings also can help parents work with their children to develop the confidence and skills they need to negotiate peer pressure. Additionally, congregational leaders and family members can work toward creating an environment that promotes avoiding use of alcohol, tobacco, and illegal and prescription drugs. It is interesting to note that studies have found that children who are involved in religious institutions are less likely to use substances (alcohol, cigarettes, marijuana, and other drugs) in adolescence, but this should not be interpreted as meaning that adolescents in religious organizations are immune to substance use. They still face many of the same situations and pressures as their peers who are not involved in a religious congregation.

One of the most important objectives with respect to adolescent substance use is to identify and address the problem as soon as possible so that the adolescent can obtain professional help and the family can get the education and support it needs. Having open conversations with adolescents in which the subject is approached seriously yet calmly can help identify problems before they become more serious. To use the analogy from the NIDA, slowing down a car going 10 mph is a lot easier than slowing down a car going 70 mph.

Suggestions for Congregational Programs

Raise awareness about substance use disorders. Raising awareness is important, as it may help overcome any stigma or misunderstandings regarding substance abuse. SAMHSA has a division focused on Faith-Based and Community Initiatives, and it has information that can be helpful to clergy and lay leaders interested in addressing substance use in the congregation and community. More information can be found on our website (www.hopkins medicine.org/jhbmc/building-hcp).

Hold open meetings to discuss substance use disorders. Open conversation is very important for both the prevention and treatment of adolescent substance use disorders. Leaders can work with members of a congregation to reduce the stigma that exists around substance use disorders. Reframing substance use disorders as a disease or illness and not a moral flaw is an important step that can take away some of the stigma and encourage treatment. No one strategy works to prevent an adolescent from substance use, but we do know that conversations with adolescents and their parents about the dangers of substance use disorders can be helpful in reducing their risk of these disorders.

Consider organizing a congregational lending library with parenting materials. This could be housed in a congregational facility or offered as a web-based resource center. Resources for this library can be found on the following websites:

www.teens.drugabuse.gov/
www.healthychildren.org/english/ages-stages/teen/substance-abuse/pag
    es/default.aspx
www.healthychildren.org/spanish/ages-stages/teen/substance-abuse/pag
    inas/default.aspx

Injuries

Childhood injuries are a major health concern, with millions of children treated in hospital emergency departments each year. Many of these injuries occur in the home, while others occur during sporting or recreational activities, and still others when children are in motor vehicles. Learning effective prevention strategies and using appropriate safety equipment can greatly reduce the risk of many of these injuries and in some cases can even result in saving lives.

The Healthy Children website sponsored by the American Academy of Pediatrics has a section on "Safety and Prevention" that offers helpful advice on preventive measures for most of the situations where childhood injuries occur. For example, to prevent accidents and injuries in the home, there is advice on dozens of topics, including high chair safety, bathroom safety tips, choking hazards, toy safety, fireplace safety, kitchen safety, preventing furniture and television tip-overs, and household chemicals. Topics on recreational safety include, among many others, bicycle safety, skateboard safety, sun safety, keeping children safe in and around pools, and safety on the playground. There is also information on preventing sports injuries. Among the topics covered are baseball strength training and injury prevention, swimming, diving, figure skating, football, ice hockey, lacrosse, martial arts, and wrestling. Information on car seats and car seat installation, booster seats, and seat belts for older children and teens is also provided. The Healthy Children website information on home, recreational, and motor vehicle safety is offered in both English (www.healthychildren.org/english/safety-preven tion/pages/default.aspx) and Spanish (www.healthychildren.org/spanish /safety-prevention/paginas/default.aspx), as is the information on preventing sports injuries (www.healthychildren.org/english/healthy-living /sports/pages/default.aspx; www.healthychildren.org/spanish/healthy-liv ing/sports/paginas/default.aspx).

Suggestions for Congregational Programs

Hold a car seat training session for families. Invite families, especially first-time parents, to see how to properly install car seats in their respective automobiles. Also, provide information on when to upgrade car seats depending on a child's size and age. Helpful safety tips for the home (e.g., childproofing your home, recognizing choking hazards, preventing furniture tip-overs) could also be shared at these sessions

Sponsor a sports and recreation day to emphasize sports safety. Talk to children and their parents about the importance of safety equipment, such as helmets and pads, as well as what to do with minor sports injuries.

Other Child and Adolescent Health Issues

Two other common health issues for children and adolescents are covered in other chapters: asthma in chapter 8 and vaccinations in chapter 15.

Examples of Congregational Programs

Father Constantine (Dean) Moralis of the Greek Orthodox Cathedral of the Annunciation in Baltimore invited an internal medicine physician to discuss substance abuse during the annual youth retreat. The conversation was held as a round table, with the physician first introducing brief facts about the rate of substance abuse in the local community and a few firsthand patient stories about the impact of substance abuse on health. Then the group (22 total, ages ranging from 14 to 19) discussed their attitudes, beliefs, and feelings toward substance abuse. The environment was one of freedom to discuss such thoughts without judgment or criticism. Further, the physician made it clear that these adolescents and young adults could do a good deed by helping friends and colleagues seek help. At the end of the 90-minute session, all those present pledged to lead a healthy life moving forward and to also see if they could help others struggling with substance abuse.

During an annual resource fair at St. John's African Methodist Episcopal Church, physicians and nurses were invited to speak to the youth regarding exercise and safety. The physicians discussed the benefits of exercise, specifically how it can help offset childhood obesity. The nurses discussed how to be safe during exercise and while engaging in sports, touching on themes of wearing proper safety equipment for certain sports, the importance of padding for joints, and how to stay adequately hydrated. Parents were also invited to sit in during the conversation, as well as ask questions. Many of the parents' concerns were focused on injuries, such as traumatic brain injury and concussions. All questions and concerns were answered thoroughly during the hour-long presentation, with handouts given at the end. The handouts included a calendar for families to list how their children would achieve 60 minutes a day of exercise. Before leaving, the health care providers asked all parents to come up with a plan for the next two days of how their children were going to exercise. All 14 families represented at the session took part in the closing activity, sharing events from "taking a long walk" to "having a family basketball game."

15

Vaccinations

It has been recognized for several hundred years that exposure to an infectious disease can make one immune from getting the same disease in the future. In particular, for most of the twentieth century, everyone knew that if you had a childhood illness such as chicken pox, that you could not catch it again. Starting in the 1950s, with the polio vaccine, there was widespread recognition that the transmission of some quite serious human diseases could be all but eliminated, and childhood polio was virtually eliminated in the United States in only a few years. Similarly, by the 1970s, with great international effort, smallpox was eliminated from the entire world. Childhood vaccinations are now routinely given to prevent a number of diseases, and in the last few decades, a number of vaccines have also been developed to prevent illness, and even death, in older adults. For example, besides the normal childhood vaccinations, it is recommended that everyone get influenza vaccine each fall, and for adults over 60, the pneumococcal vaccine and vaccine for shingles (a late-life complication related to having chicken pox as a child) are beneficial.

Vaccines are now part of a healthy individual's life from birth to old age.

So, vaccines are now part of a healthy individual's life from birth to old age. Vaccines help infants and toddlers acquire immunity to otherwise lethal infections, such as measles, tetanus, and diphtheria, and are initiated as early as two months after birth. In adults and the elderly, vaccines help boost the immune system, fighting off bacteria that cause pneumonia and viruses that cause the flu. Some vaccines may have to be given again, in order to "reboot" the immune system. An immune system's memory may decline over time, so vaccines such as tetanus require a "booster" dose. The influenza vaccine is unique among vaccines, as it is given annually because the influenza virus mutates (or changes) constantly.[1] So, each year's vaccine supply is engineered to create immunity to a few types of the virus judged most likely to be circulating in the upcoming flu season.

The Risk of Failing to Be Vaccinated

Available vaccines are intended to prevent significant injury from an infection, as well as the most serious complication of an infection—death. Even with antibiotics, which are intended to kill the bacteria that cause an active infection, many of the vaccine-preventable diseases can cause significant morbidity. This is why vaccines are so important for children, especially infants and toddlers, who are still growing and developing rapidly. Serious infections can injure growing organs, with the potential to result in lifelong complications and disability. For example, *Bordetella pertussis*, the bacteria that causes "whooping cough," may cause a toddler, whose lungs are still developing and growing, significant lung injury, resulting in poorly developed parts of the lung that will persist into adulthood.

Influenza vaccinations and the "pneumonia" vaccine (which is intended for the bacteria *Streptococcus pneumoniae*, a common cause of pneumonia) are important to obtain as adults, especially for high-risk populations, such as those with HIV infection and adults over 60. As mentioned earlier, the most effective way to manage infections, including the flu (influenza is the virus that causes "flu") and pneumonia, is to prevent them from occurring. Both of these infections are dangerous and leading causes of death in high-risk populations.

Childhood vaccinations and adult vaccinations have specific guidelines for when to obtain them.[2] However, some vaccines have restrictions because of the agent that is in them. For example, the influenza vaccine given nasally has a live virus. This live virus is harmless in persons with a normal immune system but should not be given to people with weakened immune systems. Therefore, before obtaining any vaccines, especially live virus vaccines, tell your health care provider if you live with anyone with a weak immune system (e.g., an infant, someone with HIV infection, on immunosuppressant drugs or undergoing chemotherapy, or older adults). Individuals should have conversations with their respective health care provider to assure the proper timing of vaccines, as well as the safety of the vaccine and its recipient.

In spite of the demonstrated effectiveness of vaccines, an alarming development is that **compliance** with receiving vaccinations has decreased in the pediatric population. In the early 2000s, measles was at its lowest rate of incidence ever recorded, but avoidance of this vaccine in recent years has led to a resurgence of measles. And we see that large numbers of adults (up to 40 percent of Medicare beneficiaries) do not take advantage of vaccines that can prevent serious illnesses, hospitalizations, and even death.

Research has not found any connection between autism and childhood vaccines.

One issue that has impacted the use of childhood vaccines is the controversy over vaccines and autism. The original study suggesting an association has been shown to be false, undergoing retraction by the medical journal that published it (the most extreme measure the medical community can take toward a fraudulent study). Research has not found any connection between autism and childhood vaccines.

What Can Be Done to Improve Use of Vaccinations?

Medical establishments and local and federal governments have attempted to remove certain barriers, such as access and economic concerns, that may keep persons from obtaining childhood and adult vaccines. This is important, as vaccinations can be viewed as an investment for the future well-being of persons and their communities.

One of the reasons for the declining rate of childhood vaccinations and the reluctance of many adults to get vaccinated appears to be erroneous beliefs. For example, people often believe that influenza is not a serious illness, though it leads to thousands of deaths each year. Or they think that childhood vaccinations are linked with autism, even though there is absolutely no scientific proof of this connection. Therefore, campaigns that focus on education and informing the community are necessary to ensure persons obtain appropriate vaccinations.

Vaccines are highly important for childhood development, since preventing disease will allow children to achieve their greatest healthy potential and enter adulthood without injuries from childhood infections. As for adults, certain populations must have influenza vaccinations annually (health care personnel, people over the age of 18 with chronic medical conditions, and people of any age who live or work with or care for members of high-risk groups and could easily transmit influenza). The Advisory Committee on Immunization Practices recommends that all adults who want to reduce their risk of becoming ill with influenza or of transmitting influenza to others should be vaccinated. This will also help prevent missed days of school and work, which carry their own educational and financial consequences.

Suggestions for Congregational Programs

Raise awareness about childhood vaccinations. Raising awareness of parents and soon-to-become parents about the importance of childhood vaccinations is an important step in ensuring congregational members have their children vaccinated. Places to receive vaccinations, as well as discussions of costs and insurance, should be a part of these vaccine programs, as they could be a concern for parents.

Provide information on times and places for receiving certain adult vaccinations. Certain organizations (e.g., health departments, pharmacies) may offer influenza vaccines, pneumonia vaccines, and shingles vaccines. Information regarding times and places can be obtained from local pharmacies, hospitals, and public health departments.

Hold an influenza vaccination event. Having a "flu vaccine drive" at a local congregation offers the ability to vaccinate members of the community who often have trouble accessing typical vaccination sites. Your public health department or local hospital may be able to provide personnel and supplies.

Use congregational bulletins and mailings to share information about the serious health consequences of not obtaining vaccinations. Sharing such information can help empower congregational members and motivate them to seek out proper vaccinations for children and adults.

Develop an outreach program to provide logistical support to a health care agency in order to encourage vaccination among underserved and marginalized groups. This will assure that all members of a community have an opportunity to receive the benefits of vaccinations.

Examples of Congregational Programs

Working with Southern Baptist Church of Baltimore, we coordinated a "flu shot" vaccination campaign that provided free vaccinations after Sunday worship services. The campaign required several partnerships for success: partnering with the local health commissioner's office in order to provide information on influenza, a local pharmacy to provide vaccines, and physicians from Medicine for the Greater Good (a Johns Hopkins Bayview Medical Center initiative focused on medical education and addressing health disparities). The physicians, one an infectious disease doctor and the other a pulmonary physician, spoke at the worship service. They described how the vaccine protects against the flu, and they directly addressed some of the misconceptions about vaccine. After the worship service, the congregation's pastor, Reverend Dr. Donté Hickman, reemphasized the significance of receiving the flu vaccine, encouraging his congregation to receive the vaccine that Sunday. Leading by example, Reverend Hickman and his wife both received the vaccine that day. The success of the program can be seen in surveys the congregation members took prior to receiving their flu vaccine, where over 75 percent of them reported they were not vaccinated the year prior and only received the flu vaccine this year because it was available at their congregation.

Working with a lay health educator from St. Matthew United Methodist Church in Turner Station, Maryland, to raise awareness about childhood vaccines, Medicine for the Greater Good held an initiative with a local elementary school near the church. This "Coffee with the Doctor" session was held on a weekday during drop-off time. Parents were invited to a breakfast and coffee after drop-off, as well as a discussion with a pediatric physician about vaccines. The physician spent 15 minutes highlighting what a vaccine is, what are vaccine-preventable diseases, and the recommended timeline to receive childhood vaccines. After the presentation, there was a question-and-answer session. Parents voiced their concerns, allowing the physician to reassure them by referencing current evidence to separate fact from fiction. Over 100 parents attended, in part because the event was promoted extensively at St. Matthew United Methodist Church. This is a great example of how a congregation can partner with other local organizations, such as schools, to deliver an important health message to a larger community audience.

Information Resources

Hospitals, home health agencies, public health departments, and local pharmacies are excellent local resources for programs on vaccinations, especially influenza and pneumonia vaccines. Often these organizations may sponsor annual influenza vaccination campaigns, welcoming participants from the community.

For information regarding influenza, pneumonia, and other diseases where vaccines are warranted, the Centers for Disease Control and Prevention (www.cdc.gov/vaccines) is a good resource that can provide much of the information and materials one needs for vaccine programs.

Additional information on vaccines can be found at these websites:

www.niaid.nih.gov/research/vaccines (National Institute of Allergy and
    Infectious Diseases)
www.lung.org (American Lung Association—this website helps one find
    local organizations offering influenza and pneumonia vaccines)
www.healthychildren.org/english/safety-prevention/immunizations
    /pages/default.aspx (American Academy of Pediatrics)

For more information and resources, along with additional examples of congregational health programs, please visit the book's website at www .hopkinsmedicine.org/jhbmc/building-hcp.

16

Advance Directives

The ethical basis for preparing an advance directive regarding health care is the moral and legal right of every adult to accept or refuse recommended medical treatments. Each individual can decide what medical care to accept and what to reject. Physicians, hospitals, and nursing homes must respect the wishes of competent adults, even if they disagree with certain decisions. Some people may decide that they do not want to accept a medical treatment or be on a type of life support system if they have a terminal or progressive illness and functional or cognitive disabilities, while others in similar situations may want to make sure that such treatments are continued.

If an injury or illness prevents a person from making decisions or communicating wishes, however, the situation may become far more complicated. Often the hardest decisions about life-sustaining or invasive treatments must be made by others, usually family members, who may not know whether their loved one would or would not want treatment. Therefore, it is advisable for adults of all ages to do some advance planning and use one or more advance directives to convey their wishes and decisions. The two most common ways for a person to provide guidance are to leave specific instructions, often called a living will, or to designate and authorize someone to make medical decisions in the event of incapacity.

A living will is a document that allows you to specify which treatments you would or would not want if you become incapacitated (i.e., unable to speak for yourself). The authority of a living will is limited: in most states, living wills apply only to people who have a terminal illness. In some other states, a persistent vegetative state (a neurologic diagnosis when an individual can breathe independently and appears to have sleep-wake cycles but has no evidence of consciousness) is also a "qualifying condition." For example, you can direct that you not be put on a ventilator if you are incapacitated and terminally ill or in a persistent vegetative state. If you have severe dementia and face the same decision, however, a living will would not be legally relevant in most states.

Because it is difficult to anticipate all the medical conditions you might encounter or all the treatments that might be available, and because living wills are so limited, it is important for you to designate a person to make decisions on your behalf if you cannot speak for yourself. Depending on the individual state law or regulation, such a tool is called a durable power of attorney for health care, a **health care agent**, or any of several other names. This document does not require that you be terminally ill or in a persistent vegetative state for the named individual to make medical decisions for you, only that you be incapacitated and unable to make or communicate your own decisions. Therefore, it is more broadly applicable than a living will.

Designating a substitute decision maker has an additional benefit. If the substitute agrees to act on your behalf, she or he must try to determine what *you* would have chosen if you could have foreseen your current situation. So the doctor would not say to her or him, "Do you think we should stop treatment for your loved one?" Instead, the doctor should say, "What do you think your loved one would tell us to do if she could be fully here with us for just a moment?" This is comforting to many family members, especially adult children, who do not want to feel somehow responsible for a parent's death. Further, designation of an agent does not require patients to imagine some number of awful things that could happen to them, as completing a living will does.

Federal regulations require hospitals and nursing homes to provide patients with information about advance directives and to give them an opportunity to complete these documents, often upon admission. However, attempting to fill out an advance directive during a hospital or nursing home admission is challenging, given the stressful nature of that moment. It is not the best time to consider such significant health matters carefully and make important decisions. It is difficult for patients to gather all the information about the various medical circumstances they may encounter, carefully weigh their options, and then communicate their wishes and desires to their family and physician at the time of admission. Ideally, these matters should be investigated and the documents completed at a time when a person is not so ill as to require admission to a hospital or nursing home. Also, these documents can be revised later as needed.

"Do not resuscitate" orders can also be a part of advance medical planning. These orders, placed in a hospital or nursing home chart, inform the staff that the patient does not wish to undergo attempted cardiopulmonary resuscitation (also known as CPR) if he or she experiences cardiac arrest. In some jurisdictions, individuals keep "do not resuscitate" directives in their homes so that those responding to a 911 call for emergency care do not initiate unwanted interventions. Patients' health care providers may provide them with additional information and advice about this subject.

As individuals consider some of these important issues and decisions about medical care, they may find it helpful to learn more about palliative care and hospice care. Information on both topics is provided in chapter 24 and on the book's website (www.hopkinsmedicine.org/jhbmc/building-hcp).

The Risk of Failing to Use Advance Directives

People who fail to use advance directives run the risk of receiving treatment or medical care that they would not have wanted and perhaps of being kept alive under conditions they would not find acceptable. Further, major decisions about their medical care could be made by individuals who have different values and expectations.

The absence of advance planning can also result in painful and destructive conflicts among family members. One member of the family may feel strongly that the patient would not want to be kept on life support systems, whereas another family member may feel equally strongly that it would be wrong to withdraw support. When there is conflict and the patient has not completed a living will or designated a substitute decision maker, the health care facility and doctor may need to choose a decision maker from a predetermined list of relatives. Legal involvement becomes more likely, and the decision that is ultimately made may not reflect the patient's wishes.

Two examples of the challenging medical situations that may confront individuals and the value of having completed advance directives are provided below. Both are from the experiences of co-author Dr. Panagis Galiatsatos, a pulmonary and critical care physician at Johns Hopkins.

A 29-year-old man with advanced leukemia had undergone his second bone marrow transplant four months previously. He was admitted to the intensive care unit, placed on a mechanical ventilator for breathing, and on the third day after admission his kidneys began to fail. His wife, the designated health care agent chosen by him, wanted to fight on. However, she showed the staff that in his advance directive he stated that he wished to be allowed to pass peacefully, without suffering, if there were no way of curing his current condition and restoring an acceptable quality of life. The physicians, the nurses, and the man's family all agreed that, given his incurable condition, it was appropriate to begin to focus on comfort care and to withdraw the invasive machinery, and he died peacefully. His wife was contacted a few months later, and although she continued to grieve, she said that she had no regrets or guilt because she knew she had followed her husband's wishes.

A 72-year-old woman was admitted from home for pneumonia. In the emergency room, she was put on a mechanical ventilator to support her breathing. Unfortunately, her critical illness left her unable to communicate. Her husband had died a few years previously, and she had no advance directives, so it became the responsibility of her three children, all of whom lived out of state, to make decisions about her care. It was evident that the stress of knowing their mother was critically ill was matched by the stress they felt because they could not agree on what their mother would have wanted in this situation. Several meetings followed with health care providers in order to reach a compromised consensus between the siblings on how to approach their mother's critical situation.

What Can Be Done to Prevent Loss of Control Over Medical Decisions?

Most people are aware of advance directives—at least living wills—and say they are in favor of using them. However, surveys show that few adults have formally expressed their wishes and completed appropriate forms. One reason that people fail to complete the forms is that both health care providers and patients are reluctant to broach the subject. Therefore, it is important to encourage people to discuss this matter with their health care providers and not to wait for their providers to take the initiative.

One misconception people often have is that they must have an attorney prepare a living will or a durable power of attorney for health care (health care agent) and thus are reluctant to incur the costs associated with hiring legal counsel. Fortunately, establishing advance directives does not require the services of an attorney. Forms can be obtained from hospitals, home health agencies, and several national organizations. Further, the forms obtained from these organizations can be modified to suit each person's wishes. Another option is for people to write their own advance directives. These are legal and acceptable directives as long as they are properly witnessed by two adults, only one of whom may be a member of the immediate family and neither of whom may be designated as the surrogate (substitute) decision maker. They are, however, subject to the same restrictions as the more formal documents.

Another misconception held by some people is that they will permanently lose control of decisions about their medical care once a living will or durable power of attorney for health care has been prepared and signed. They think they are signing a document that is irrevocable. However, these documents are used only when patients are unable to communicate their wishes. People can change or revoke an advance directive at any time, including naming another individual to be the health care agent.

People need to be encouraged to discuss their wishes and feelings about end-of-life matters with family members or other designated decision makers. These individuals need to know that the documents exist and that they were executed after careful consideration of the medical circumstances and options. A statement or declaration of personal values completed by the patient can be helpful to family members who need to understand the patient's wishes and decisions. Additionally, a statement of values can serve as a useful guide for a person who has the durable power of attorney for health care.

Suggestions for Congregational Programs

Sponsor a program on advance directives. Hold a program where a physician, nurse, or social worker explains advance directives, going over medical circumstances patients may encounter and discussing the medical decisions they might face. Forms to distribute at these programs can be obtained from the websites listed at the end of this chapter or from local hospitals and home health agencies.

Sponsor a program on ethical decision making. This could be led by clergy and could include examples of statements or declarations of values.

Arrange for members of your congregation to make audio or video recordings of their wishes and instructions on end-of-life matters. These could then be used to supplement written documents if the situation arises.

Examples of Congregational Programs

During a Shabbat service at Temple Beth El in Ormond Beach, Florida, Rabbi Barry Altman asked the members to stay after the service to hear brief presentations on advance directives by Dr. Alvin Smith, a well-known oncologist (who was not a member of the congregation), and Marshall Barkin, an attorney (who was a member). Dr. Smith offered several examples of situations in which patients with terminal illnesses who had lost their ability to communicate with others were forced to receive medical treatment they probably did not want. However, because they had not prepared advance directives expressing their wishes, the doctor and hospital were forced to continue the treatment. He strongly urged members of the congregation to avoid these situations by completing a living will and designating a trusted individual as their surrogate decision maker. Mr. Barkin provided additional information about these documents and further encouraged members to use them. Rabbi Altman then reinforced their advice by also recommending that members take these measures to ensure that their wishes about end-of-life care would be honored.

Another example is an advance directive initiative held over the Easter season at Southern Baptist Church in Baltimore. Information on advance directives was given at worship services every Sunday for a month, with commentary provided by the congregation's spiritual leader, Dr. Donté Hickman, who highlighted the importance of having, at a minimum, "someone to speak for you." Additionally, pledge cards asking adults in the congregation to make a commitment to designate a health care agent were handed out. By the Sunday after Easter, 169 cards had been returned, with 100 pledging to identify a health care agent, and 69 indicating they already had identified and designated an agent. Pleased with the success of this important initiative, Dr. Hickman promised to offer this program again the following year.

Information Resources

Hospitals, home health agencies, and health care clinics can provide copies of advance directives, and they also may be able to provide speakers for congregational programs. There also may be attorneys interested in volunteering their time to speak to groups about advance directives.

Several national organizations provide information and materials on advance directives. These include:

Aging with Dignity (www.agingwithdignity.org)
Caring Connections (www.caringinfo.org)

For more information and resources, along with additional examples of congregational health programs, please visit the book's website at www .hopkinsmedicine.org/jhbmc/building-hcp.

17

Communicating with
Health Care Providers

Good, clear communication between patients and their health care providers is absolutely essential, but many people have had the experience of coming out of an appointment feeling more confused than when they went in. It is not unusual for people to report that they do not fully understand their illness or what they should do to manage their condition effectively, even though they have had several meetings with their health care provider. There are a number of factors that can contribute to this confusion and uncertainty. Some of the obstacles patients frequently mention include:

Medical terminology: "My doctor acted like I should understand the terminology he was using. I would have felt stupid telling him I didn't."

Doctor's schedule: "My doctor seemed too busy to discuss all of my concerns. She looked rushed, and there were so many other patients in her waiting room."

Anxiety: "I was so nervous about my situation that I forgot to tell him something important."

Attitude toward medical professionals: "I find it difficult to question or be assertive with my health care provider. It's easier to just listen quietly."

Provider's interview style: "His questions led me away from some of the things I had intended to discuss. I never got back to several of my concerns."

Information overload: "There was just too much information. I was overwhelmed."

Problems with memory: "I understood what she said, but by the time I got home, I had forgotten most of it."

These and other problems can interfere with the exchange of clear, accurate information between patients and their health care providers. Without good communication, the medical encounter cannot reach its full potential and may, in some cases, even create new problems. Physicians and other health professionals need accurate information from patients if they are to arrive at a correct diagnosis and develop the right treatment plan, and patients need information about their condition and recommended treatment that is clear and easy to understand if the treatment plan is going to be successful.

Although many factors can contribute to the problem of poor communication between patients and providers, patients can use a few key strategies to overcome these obstacles, and the benefits of adopting these strategies are well established. People who take the initiative to improve communication with their providers receive more factual information from their providers, are more likely to follow through with treatment recommendations, and report greater satisfaction with the care they are receiving.

Patients who take the initiative to improve communication with their providers receive more factual information from their providers and report greater satisfaction with the care they are receiving.

A key point for patients to remember as they prepare for medical visits is that most important issues can be covered during a meeting with a provider if the information is well organized and presented in a direct, clear manner. Health care providers are trained to take in and process large amounts of information in a relatively brief period of time. The key to a successful, productive meeting with a provider—one where all major concerns are shared and all important questions are asked—is for the patient to have a well-organized, carefully prepared list that covers all the important items he or she wishes to discuss.

We have written a brief guide, *Making the Most of Your Medical Visit*, that individuals can use as they prepare for their medical visits and during their meetings with doctors and other health care providers. It also has advice and suggestions that address some of the concerns that often emerge after patients have left their provider's office. This guide can be copied and distributed to interested persons. It also is available in PDF format on our website (www.hopkinsmedicine.org/jhbmc/building-hcp).

Making the Most of Your Medical Visit

Preparing for Your Medical Visit

One of the best ways to show your health care provider that you want to be an active and informed participant in your health care is to take with you to your appointment some basic information about your medical situation along with a list of three or four questions that you would like answered. Be sure to let your provider know at the beginning of the visit that you have this information, as well as several questions you want to cover. This will show that you have given thought to the medical issues of greatest concern to you and that you want to make good use of your time together. It is a good idea to write your questions on a card or sheet of paper in case your provider's answer to one of your questions shifts your attention away from your other concerns.

Below are a number of questions that can help you organize this information and prepare for your appointment.

What is your "number one" concern? What problem or problems do you want addressed? For example, is your primary objective to have your condition diagnosed and treated as aggressively as possible, or do you want to find a treatment that minimizes pain and allows you to continue with activities you enjoy? Sometimes physicians and other providers are so focused on identifying and treating the underlying disease that they do not pay enough attention to aspects of the disease or treatments that are of greatest concern to patients.

What symptoms are you experiencing? Be as specific as possible. When did they begin? If they are not constant, then at what times or in what situations do they occur? What makes them improve or become worse? Have you ever had these symptoms before? If so, how long ago and how were they treated? How is this illness affecting your day-to-day life?

What is your understanding of the problem? Perhaps you have discussed your problem with a friend or looked for information on the Internet. (Many of the health-related websites are excellent, but there also are many that are not reliable. Chapter 25 lists some of the most reliable websites.) If you have some ideas about what you are experiencing or what has caused the problem, share these with your provider.

What remedies have you already tried? Have you taken any over-the-counter medications? Have you changed your diet or any of your habits in an attempt to address the problem? If so, did your efforts help?

Are you being treated for any other problems by another health care professional? If so, who are you seeing and for what problems?

What medications, including nonprescription medications and nutritional supplements, are you currently taking? Often the best way to provide this information is for you to carry all your medications with you to your appointment.

Have there been any significant changes in your life since your last appointment (e.g., illness or death of a loved one, difficulties in relationships with family or friends, new living arrangements, change in finances, new responsibilities at home or at work, change in your ability to handle household matters)?

How have you been feeling emotionally lately? Have you felt anxious or depressed about your health or anything else going on in your life?

Are there any potential obstacles to the treatment or additional diagnostic tests that might be recommended (e.g., financial limitations, family or work responsibilities)?

Have you completed any advance directives (e.g., living will, health care agent, or durable power of attorney for health care)? If so, be sure to take copies with you and ask your provider to add them to your chart. If not, then consider discussing these with your provider. More information about advance directives can be found in chapter 16.

One more step you should consider as you prepare for your medical visit is to ask a family member or friend to go with you. If you think it might be difficult for you to present all the information that needs to be presented or to ask important questions or to remember what is recommended, then ask someone to go with you to your appointment.

Meeting with Your Provider

Remember to take your basic medical information and your questions with you, along with paper and pen to record the information and recommendations your provider will be giving you. Also, carry all your medications, both prescription and nonprescription, or at least a detailed list of these medications. If you are having someone go with you, be sure to let them know exactly what role you want him or her to play during your visit.

If a nurse or medical assistant takes your blood pressure before you see your provider, ask for the results and record these. Later, during your examination, ask your provider what he or she thinks about your blood pressure.

When your provider arrives and begins questioning you, start by explaining your number one reason for the visit, being as specific as you can about your symptoms, concerns, and hopes. Also be sure to mention that you have several questions you need to ask before you leave.

When sharing information about your symptoms and what you believe they may indicate, be as specific, complete, and organized as possible. Exactly what are you experiencing now and how does that differ from what you normally experience? If some symptoms suggest to you a certain diagnosis, perhaps based on what someone else told you or what you found on the Internet or in a medical book, then report those symptoms and ask if they might be an indication of a particular condition. For example, if you have had difficulty sleeping, have lost weight, and no longer enjoy activities you previously found pleasurable, and you have heard that these might be an indication of depression, share this information and ask if this means you might, indeed, be depressed. This will enable your provider to ask key questions and determine if that is the correct diagnosis.

If you believe that your medical problem might be related to stress you are experiencing or something you have done, share this with your provider. If you are concerned that this information would prove embarrassing if family members or friends were to learn about it, ask your provider exactly how he or she handles information that you want to be kept in confidence. Part of a federal law, the Privacy Rule of the **Health Insurance Portability and Accountability Act (HIPAA)**, strictly limits what information health care professionals can share with or tell others—even a spouse—without a patient's permission.

If your provider does not ask if you are seeing any other health professionals or receiving treatment for other problems, go ahead and volunteer this information. Be sure to include treatments that may not be strictly medical (e.g., acupuncture, nutritional or herbal supplements, chiropractic care, homeopathy). Also, let your provider know about the medications, prescription and nonprescription, that you are taking.

As your provider conducts a physical examination, do not be reluctant to ask if he or she has found anything of importance. Did your heart sound okay? What about your lungs? If he or she seems to spend more time on one part of the examination, ask why. And this would be a good time to ask about your blood pressure.

Following the physical examination and your report of your symptoms, concerns, medications, and other medical problems for which you are being treated, your provider may be able to give you a diagnosis. Your diagnosis should be given in terms that you understand. If you do not understand the terms being used, do not hesitate to speak up and ask for clarification. In fact, even if you are relatively confident that you understand the diagnosis, it is a good idea to repeat it and to put into your own words your understanding of the condition. We recommend that you or the person who has accompanied you to your appointment write down the diagnosis and explanation and then ask your provider to read over what has been written to be sure that it is correct.

If for any reason you do not believe that the diagnosis you have been given is correct or that the treatment recommended for you will be effective, voice your doubts to your provider and explain why you disagree. It is far better to politely and respectfully express your doubts during the appointment than to keep your thoughts to yourself and then, once you leave your appointment, disregard your provider's opinion and recommendations.

It is usually a good idea to ask what has caused your condition or what factors have contributed to its development. For many chronic conditions, there is more than one contributing factor, so it may be difficult for your provider to give a definitive answer to this question, but he or she should be able to provide you with a general explanation. Here again, we recommend that you repeat and then write down this information.

Once the diagnosis has been determined and contributing factors discussed, your provider will offer treatment recommendations. Often this will include a prescription for one or more medications. It is important that you understand exactly what is being prescribed and why it is being prescribed. Estimates are that as many as 50 percent or more of patients do not take their medications appropriately. Frequently this is because of a breakdown in communication between provider and patient.

If your provider does not volunteer enough information about the medication, you need to ask a number of questions. Exactly what are the expected benefits of the medication? How long will it take for you to notice the benefits? How should it be taken? Is this medication likely to interfere with any of your other medications? Is this a medication that will need to be taken only for a limited period of time, or is it likely that you will need to remain on it indefinitely? Is it possible that you will experience some side effects? If so, what should you do? Be sure to write down the answers to these questions and review your notes with your provider before you leave.

If there is any reason why you might not be able to take the medication you have been prescribed, do not hesitate to mention this to your provider. Doctors and other health care providers understand and appreciate the fact that the latest and best medication for a particular medical condition is of no value if it is not taken as prescribed. If the cost of the medication is the obstacle, explain this to your provider. Often a less expensive alternative that has similar benefits can be prescribed. If your work schedule or other aspects of your life would make it difficult for you to take the medication at the times prescribed, ask if there is a similar medication that would be a better fit with your daily routine.

It is possible your provider will determine that what are generally referred to as lifestyle factors are contributing to your condition and need to be modified. This recommendation often presents at least two challenges for patients. First, many patients do not think of a change in physical activity or diet as a *medical* treatment. To them, this type of recommendation does not seem to be as important as a recommendation to take a prescribed medication. Therefore, it is important that you have a clear understanding of the connection between these lifestyle factors and your condition. How will a change in your behavior—what you eat or your level of physical activity—affect your medical condition? What will happen if you do not make the recommended changes?

Second, even when patients understand the connection between certain lifestyle factors and their condition, it can be difficult to modify habits that are deeply ingrained and often highly pleasurable. Patients need to recognize this and ask for help implementing and maintaining the recommended changes. For some problems (e.g., smoking), your provider may be able to prescribe medication that will help. If the problem with the recommended modification (e.g., adopting a low-fat diet) is that family members are unlikely to cooperate and support your efforts to change, ask if your provider would be willing to meet with them to explain the importance of these recommendations. If you believe it would be easier for you to make the recommended changes if you could be around others who are working toward a similar goal, ask if there are any community groups or programs that are focused on the same issue (e.g., weight reduction).

Once you are clear about the diagnosis, contributing factors, and treatment recommendations (remember to ask questions if you are unclear about any of these matters), share with your provider your reaction to this information. Do you feel better now that you know the diagnosis and how your condition will be treated? Are you confident that you will be able to follow the recommendations? How has this information affected you emotionally? Has any of what you have heard frightened you or discouraged you? Are you worried that your illness or the treatments are going to limit your ability to work or continue with other activities you value and enjoy? If you find that you are pessimistic about your ability to carry out the treatment recommendations or feel overwhelmed emotionally by what you have heard, ask your provider for suggestions about a support group or a mental health professional who could help you.

For certain illnesses, you may want to address other issues during a visit with your provider. If you believe that your illness is likely to progress (e.g., Parkinson's disease, multiple sclerosis), even with the recommended treatment, you may want to ask your provider about the long-term course of your illness and what this may mean with respect to your living arrangements. Would it be advisable for you to make some modifications in your house or apartment (e.g., grab rails, ramps)? Should you or family members begin looking for new living arrangements (e.g., an assisted living facility, a continuing care retirement community)? Will you need to consider a hospice program at some point? You also may want to get advice about what you should consider as you prepare or update advance directives (see chapter 16 for more information on advance planning).

As your visit draws to an end, be sure that you have asked all of your questions and that you understand your provider's answers. You should have a clear understanding of your diagnosis, likely contributing factors, and treatment recommendations. If you feel it would be helpful to learn more about your illness or treatment, ask if there are printed materials or a reliable book or website you could read for more information. Finally, be certain that you know when you are to return for a subsequent appointment or when and where you need to go for additional tests.

Follow-Up

The visit with your provider is certainly an essential part of good medical care. However, for most chronic conditions, what takes place at home is just as important as what takes place when meeting with your doctor or other health professionals. In fact, most of the recommended care will take place at home. For example, the medications prescribed by your provider will be of little benefit if they are not taken correctly, and sound advice about lifestyle modifications is of no value if it is not followed. Therefore, it is important for you to take the steps needed to implement treatment recommendations and to do so as soon as you can after visiting your provider.

It is not uncommon for questions about your illness and/or the treatment recommendations to arise after you have left your provider's office. You may find that the medication you were prescribed does not seem to be having the beneficial effects you were expecting or that it is producing some unpleasant side effects. Or perhaps you are no longer experiencing the symptoms that prompted your medical visit and thus are not certain that you need to continue taking your medication. Any questions about whether or not to continue taking a prescribed medication should be made in consultation with your provider. You should, at a minimum, call your provider's office and express your concerns. If you have discovered that the medication you have been prescribed is too expensive or not on the list of medications covered by your insurance policy, you may want to ask your pharmacist about alternatives and ask that he or she contact your provider to see if the prescription can be changed.

Sometimes an illness is unusual or rare and getting the opinion of another physician or specialist is appropriate. You may not necessarily understand or know when this is the case, but asking your provider whether or not a consultation with another specialist is worthwhile is always a reasonable thing to do. When exceptionally rare or life-threatening conditions are diagnosed, or if a major operation is recommended, you may be comforted by getting a second opinion concerning the recommended course of treatment. Often, it is advisable to turn to a regional or national academic medical center in these cases, and most are set up to handle these types of consultations and referrals. To prepare for such a visit, you should gather and send all appropriate medical records to the expert being consulted so that she or he is prepared to meet with you knowing as much information as possible about your condition and the concerns you want addressed (e.g., recommendations regarding treatment, need for further testing, consideration of other approaches to diagnosis and treatment).

If blood work or other tests were conducted during or shortly after your medical visit, take the initiative to check back with your provider's office (or the patient portal if your provider is using an electronic health record) to get the results and to see if you need to return for another appointment or make any changes in your treatment. Given the complexity of modern medicine, test results can be available within hours of your visit (e.g., routine blood work) or take days or even weeks for final results to be released. Particularly for radiology (e.g., X-rays, mammograms, MRIs) or pathology (e.g., skin biopsies), test results and receipt of reports can be delayed. Therefore, it is important for you to track and ensure that your provider receives the final report and that any critical information is shared with you.

Remember, good communication between patients and providers is at the heart of good medical care, and you can do your part by following these three basic recommendations:

- Be prepared for your visit with your provider. Organize key information about your medical situation and prepare several questions you would like answered.
- Be active during your appointment. Ask questions and do not hesitate to request clarification if you do not understand your provider's answers.
- Follow through on your provider's recommendations. If there is a reason you cannot, get back in touch with your provider to explore other alternatives.

The Patient Advocate or Health Partner

One of the recommendations in the guide, *Making the Most of Your Medical Visit*, is for people to ask a family member or friend to accompany them to their appointments. This can be especially important for those who have multiple chronic conditions and thus need a variety of medications or treatments. Unfortunately, some individuals do not have a family member or friend who is able to serve in this capacity. One way religious congregations can assist these individuals is to recruit and prepare volunteers to serve in this role. Working closely with health care professionals and religious leaders, we have prepared a brief guide for members of congregations who are interested in serving as **patient advocates** or health partners, helping patients prepare for medical visits, and then accompanying them to their appointments. This guide, *Serving as a Patient Advocate*, is available in PDF format on the book's website (www.hopkinsmedicine.org/jhbmc/build

ing-hcp) and can be downloaded and copied. The guide can be supplemented with the advice of an experienced physician, nurse, or other health professional familiar with the local medical community and health care system.

Suggestions for Congregational Programs

Invite a local physician who is known as a good communicator to speak on the topic of doctor-patient communication and how patients can handle difficult issues with their health care providers.

Sponsor a program on how to find reliable medical information on the Internet.

Invite a representative from your hospital to talk about medical tests commonly ordered by physicians.

Invite a primary care provider to discuss how she or he conducts physical examinations.

Invite a health care provider to lead a program on medical terminology commonly used with patients.

18

Modifying Common
Risk Factors

There are a number of risk factors for most chronic diseases, some of which are beyond our control (e.g., age, gender, family history). But there are other risk factors, often referred to as lifestyle factors, over which we can exert considerable influence. In this chapter we discuss four of these factors—stress, inadequate physical activity, excess weight, and smoking—and offer strategies for modifying them. For each lifestyle factor, we have written brief guides that can be copied and handed out to individuals interested in modifying that factor. These guides also are available in PDF format on the book's website (www.hopkinsmedicine.org/jhbmc/building-hcp) and can be downloaded and copied. Each guide is followed by suggestions for congregational programs and information about additional resources.

> There are a number of risk factors for most chronic diseases, some of which are beyond our control, but there are other risk factors over which we can exert considerable influence.

A Brief Guide to Stress Management

Stress is an inevitable part of life—there is simply no way to completely avoid it. But when it is prolonged or excessive, it can have harmful consequences for our health. For example, it can impair immune system functioning or trigger the release of hormones that speed up heart rate and raise blood pressure. Stress also can increase our risk of illness or worsen existing illnesses by making it more difficult for us to maintain a healthy lifestyle (e.g., regular exercise, nutritious diet). Therefore, it is important for us to learn how to manage stress effectively.

The first step in managing stress is to identify what is causing it. Although this might appear to be a simple assignment—you may quickly point to new responsibilities at work or a crisis with the family (or both)—it is not always clear exactly why a certain situation is stressful or what elements of the situation make it so. Two people can face the same challenging situation and yet differ dramatically in their reactions. Often it is helpful to begin by keeping a journal in which you record not only the various tasks you have each day but also your thoughts about these tasks and your ability to handle them.

- Exactly what did you do that was so stressful?
- Who else was involved?
- What was said?
- How did you feel about what you did or what was said?

It is also a good idea to keep track of the activities and experiences that you enjoyed each day and the times you were able to break free of the stressful situation and relax at least a little. Were there moments of joy and appreciation for something or someone you encountered? Perhaps you experienced a sense of awe and wonder as you watched a beautiful sunrise or looked through a book with photos of some of the world's magnificent natural wonders. Or maybe it was just an enjoyable conversation you had with someone.

The next step is to carefully analyze your daily activities and thoughts.

- Which task or tasks caused the most stress?
- Was there one particular responsibility you found stressful, or was the stress you experienced the result of having to handle too many responsibilities?
- Did the people with whom you interacted add to or reduce the stress?
- What did you say to yourself about how you handled your responsibilities?
- Did you feel you did a good job?
- Was the task as difficult or overwhelming as you had anticipated?
- How much time did you have to do some of the things that you enjoy?
- What situations or activities did you find relaxing or renewing?

Your next step depends on what you discovered through your analysis of your daily activities. Below are some typical causes of stress along with strategies for addressing each.

"I have too many responsibilities." This is a common problem, and there are different approaches to managing this source of stress. First, prioritize your various responsibilities or tasks, and then ask yourself several questions: Which are the essential tasks—the ones you absolutely must continue? Are there any that you can set aside or ask someone else to take over? Frequently we are reluctant to step back from responsibilities or hand them off to others, but there may come a time when you need to do this in order to carry out your most important responsibilities and, at the same time, maintain your own health.

Improving your time management skills also may help. Often, when new responsibilities have been added, a person's life becomes disorganized. Whereas previously you were able to handle all of your responsibilities without giving much thought to your schedule or relying on a planner, you now find that everything seems to be in disarray. It can be helpful to set aside enough time to list each day's responsibilities, establish priorities, and create a realistic plan for handling these responsibilities. And when you are filling in your planner, be sure to schedule some time for yourself! Treat this time, even if it is only for a few minutes, as a high priority item, essential to maintaining the good health you need to carry out your key responsibilities.

"Other people are expecting too much of me." Or *"I'm not getting the help that I need."* If your analysis has revealed that other people seem to have unrealistic expectations of you, or if you have found that individuals who could be assisting you are not doing so, then it may be helpful to work on improving your communication skills. This is not to say that you have poor communication skills but that new circumstances may call for a change in your approach.

Chances are that at least some of the people with whom you interact are not aware that you are feeling overwhelmed. They may not know about all of your various duties, or it may appear to them that everything is under control and that you do not need any assistance. The only way these individuals are going to come to your aid is if you take the initiative to say in a calm but assertive manner what you are feeling about your situation and needs. The best way to handle this type of communication, especially during a crisis or period of great stress, is to identify exactly what you need to say, plan how to say it, and even rehearse it a few times. And remember, the goal is to communicate what you need, not to criticize others. For example, a simple statement, "I am feeling overwhelmed and really need some help," is more effective than saying, "Everyone seems to be too busy with their own lives to help me."

"*I find negative thoughts running through my head day and night.*" What we say to ourselves about ourselves, our situation, and the future can create a tremendous amount of stress. In fact, many people find that their anticipation of what lies ahead is often more stressful than the actual tasks and that their negative thoughts intrude into parts of the day when they could be enjoying their time. If this is the case, you can work on recognizing the negative thoughts and replacing them with more realistic, positive ones. This will take practice, but it can be done. For example, instead of saying to yourself (perhaps over and over again), "I'm dreading tomorrow. I'll never be able to handle everything I'm expected to do," replace it with a more realistic statement, "I'm not looking forward to tomorrow, but I've handled days like this before and will be able to handle this one, too." And try to keep your attention on the present, not the future.

But what if a careful analysis of your daily activities reveals that there is no way for you to cut back significantly on your responsibilities or to enlist the help of others? And what if you find that most of your negative thoughts about your situation are not exaggerated or unrealistic? There still are strategies that you can employ to reduce stress. One of the most important is to find someone you can trust and in whom you can confide your feelings about the difficulties in your life—a friend, a member of the clergy, a mental health professional, or members of a support group. Often during our most stressful times we are reluctant to let others know what we are going through, but that is exactly when we need to take the initiative to reach out and ask for help. You should not try to go through any difficult period—marital strife, financial difficulties, caring for an ill family member—by yourself.

Something else to look for as you review your journal is whether or not you are still involved in activities that you find enjoyable and renewing. Often when we encounter stressful and demanding situations, the first thing we allow to drop from our schedule are activities that bring us pleasure and restore our spirits—listening to our favorite music, reading interesting books, or taking leisurely walks. Granted, you may no longer have as much time as you did before to enjoy these activities, but with careful planning you should be able to find ways to get some of these back into your life. You should not underestimate the importance of these activities. We all need these types of activities to restore and strengthen our mental health.

Relaxation exercises are another tool that individuals can use to counteract some of the effects of stress. One of the commonly used approaches is "progressive relaxation." In this method, you systematically tense different muscle groups and then gradually relax those muscles. You can start by tensing the muscles around your eyes for four or five seconds and then slowly releasing this tension until these muscles are completely relaxed. Next, tense the muscles around your mouth and jaw for a few seconds and then gradually release the tension until these muscles are relaxed. Follow this procedure for the other muscle groups, eventually moving all the way down to your feet and toes. While doing these exercises, be sure to keep your attention focused on the exercises themselves and to set aside any thoughts about your stressful situation.

It is not always easy to achieve a relaxed state when your life is full of demanding responsibilities, but it can be done. The key is to practice your relaxation procedures regularly. Therefore, it is important to carve out of your schedule each day at least 15 minutes for practice. More information about relaxation techniques and other stress management strategies can be found on our website (www.hopkinsmedicine.org/jhbmc/building-hcp) and on the MedlinePlus website listed below under Information Resources.

Suggestions for Congregational Programs
Offer classes on relaxation.
Sponsor a stress management program offered by a mental health professional.
Organize support groups or provide information about where individuals can find a support group.

Information Resources
https://medlineplus.gov/stress.html

A Brief Guide to Increasing Physical Activity

One of the major risk factors for several serious medical conditions, including heart disease, stroke, and diabetes, is physical inactivity. Despite this well-documented link, the National Center for Health Statistics has found that only a little over half of American adults meet the federal physical activity guidelines for aerobic activity through leisure-time activity (150 minutes a week of moderate-intensity aerobic activity), with African American and Hispanic/Latino adults having rates lower than non-Hispanic/Latino white adults.[1] Clearly, there is a need for more programs to educate adults about the health benefits of increased physical activity and to provide ongoing encouragement and support for maintaining regular individualized programs of exercise.

Although regular exercise is safe for most adults, even those with chronic conditions, it is always advisable to check with your health provider before embarking on a new exercise program. Once you have been medically cleared, you are ready to begin. The best way to start is to take the time to develop a plan for a program of physical activity that you will be able to enjoy and sustain for years. An important initial step is to be clear about your motivation and readiness.

- Why do you believe it is important to become more physically active?
- What are the benefits of becoming more active?
- How is your life likely to be affected if you do not increase your physical activity?
- Are you ready to make it a priority?

When identifying the benefits, think of both long-term and short-term benefits. By increasing your physical activity you are increasing the odds of preventing various medical conditions, or at least minimizing their impact, and living longer, but you also are likely to experience more immediate benefits, including greater endurance that will enable you to engage in more activities you enjoy. Increased activity is also usually associated with improved mood and a greater sense of well-being. Make a list of these benefits and refer back to it often.

Next, look back over the past few years to gain a better understanding of why you have not been active enough.

- Was there a time when you were physically active?
- What activities did you enjoy then?
- Why did you stop or decrease your activity?
- What are the obstacles that have kept you from being active recently?
- How can you overcome or work around these obstacles?

Be as specific as you can. If lack of time has been the major obstacle, what responsibilities or activities are creating the problem? Which of these can be dropped, reduced, or shifted? Can you identify times when you could substitute physical activity for a passive activity (e.g., a walk around the neighborhood instead of watching a television program)?

The next step is to select the right activity. As you consider options, it is important that you find an activity that fits your schedule, living situation, and finances. You do not have to join a fitness club or buy expensive equipment to become more physically fit. Nor do you have to become a marathon runner. For example, if you do not have easy access to exercise facilities, walking regularly around your neighborhood or in a park or on the track at a nearby school could be an option, and all that is required is a good pair of walking shoes.

- Choose an activity you enjoy. You are much more likely to be able to stick with an activity that is fun or interesting for you. If you find a particular activity difficult or boring, try another one.
- If it is easier to be physically active when you have others with you, ask a friend to join you or find a group activity, perhaps an exercise class at a recreation center.
- Develop a specific plan and write it down. Then make a commitment, in writing, to follow your plan. For example:
  - What are you going to do? Brisk walking
  - Where will you do it? In the neighborhood
  - When will you do it? In the evening, instead of watching one of my television programs
- Set reasonable, specific goals. Do not be overly ambitious at the start. Although you may want to eventually achieve the recommended goal of 150 minutes of moderate-intensity aerobic activity a week, that doesn't need to be your initial goal. For example, you can start with the goal of a 10-minute brisk walk three evenings every week, then gradually add more time and distance.
- Enlist the support of family and friends. Explain why it is important for you to begin and stay with this program. Ask for their ongoing encouragement and support.
- Keep track of your activity. A simple activity log can help you identify what is working well with your plan and where you may need to make adjustments. It also can give you a sense of accomplishment.
- Plan for interruptions, both scheduled (e.g., vacations) and unscheduled (e.g., illnesses). There is no need to feel guilty when these interruptions occur, but make a commitment to get back to your activity plan as soon as possible.

In addition to your primary plan for increasing physical activity, search for other opportunities to add some physical activity to your daily routine. For example:

- When possible, take the stairs instead of the elevator
- Use work breaks or part of your lunch break to take a walk
- Park your car farther from the store when shopping
- If you use the bus or subway, get off one or two stops before your regular one

Suggestions for Congregational Programs

Sponsor a workshop on exercise led by a physical therapist.

Organize groups into friendly competition (e.g., which group can accumulate the most distance walked during a certain period?).

Create a list for members who are looking for partners to join them in a program of regular physical activity (e.g., walking or biking together).

Organize a walking group.

Information Resources

https://www.niddk.nih.gov/health-information/health-communication-programs/win/Pages/default.aspx

A Brief Guide to Losing Weight

The most common approach to weight loss has been dieting, a method in which people focus on reducing their caloric intake. Although the basic equation underlying this approach is correct—weight loss results when the calories you use exceed the calories you take in—the weight loss produced by using this approach alone is generally not maintained for long. A more effective strategy for weight loss is a multidimensional approach that can be incorporated into your overall lifestyle and sustained for the rest of your life.

The first step is to assess your readiness to begin a weight-reduction program.

- What is your motivation for trying to lose weight?
- Are you clear about the health risks of maintaining your current weight and the benefits of losing weight?
- Have you checked with your health care provider in order to set a reasonable goal and to get advice about any specific dietary concerns?

- Have you thought about how to enlist the support of your family and friends?

The next step is to carefully monitor and record your eating habits.

- What do you eat?
- How much of each food do you eat?
- When do you eat?
- Where do you eat?
- Do you eat more when people are around or when you are by yourself?
- Are your eating habits when dining out different from those at home?
- Which setting is more challenging?

Be as specific as possible. It is also helpful to record any situations or emotions that trigger your desire to eat. For example, do you eat more when you are feeling lonely or anxious? You should plan on continuing to monitor your eating habits as you implement your weight-reduction program. This will enable you to identify new obstacles and then make appropriate adjustments.

After you have analyzed the various aspects of your eating habits, you need to take the time to begin developing a plan that addresses the problem areas you have identified. The goal is to come up with practical strategies that will make it easier for you to cut back on the calories you consume. Some possible parts of a plan may be readily apparent. For example, if you discovered that you find it hard not to snack when there are cookies or other high-calorie items in your kitchen cabinet, you should purchase fewer of these high-calorie items and more healthful, low-calorie items. (Helpful hint: Most people find it easier to pass up tasty, high-calorie items in the grocery store if they do their shopping immediately after they have had a satisfying meal. Also, make up your grocery list in advance and stick to it.) If you get hungry sometimes while working and the only food available at your worksite are high-calorie snacks, you can prepare for this by purchasing or preparing some low-calorie snacks to take with you. Or if you find that you tend to snack when you are lonely, substitute an alternative activity—perhaps calling a friend or going for a walk.

If you find that you tend to overeat when you are dining out, you can cut back on the frequency of dining out, or you can opt instead to reduce the amount of food you eat in restaurants. Although leaving food on your plate may run counter to what you learned as a child, it is an important part of losing weight, especially because the portions served by many restaurants are quite large. And there is always the option of asking for a "doggy bag" and saving part of your dinner for another meal.

Another useful strategy to employ, no matter where you are eating, is to pay more attention to the actual eating process. The goal here is to eat less but enjoy it more. One way to do this is to eat more slowly and focus on savoring each bite or mouthful, enjoying the taste and texture of your food. Record how long it typically takes you to eat your meal and then work on gradually lengthening this period. If you find it difficult to eat more slowly, try putting down your eating utensils after every few mouthfuls. This generally slows eating and reduces the total amount of food consumed.

Physical activity needs to be a part of your weight-reduction plan. This can take many forms—walking, biking, jogging, swimming, aerobic exercise classes, and so on. The best strategy is to choose an activity you enjoy and then add it to your daily routine. Most experts recommend 30 minutes of moderate-intensity physical activity five or more days a week. If you find it hard to carve a 30-minute block out of your schedule, then break it down into shorter blocks of time. Three 10-minute periods devoted to physical activity burn as many calories as one 30-minute period. Another good strategy, and one that yields double benefits, is to go for a walk during a break at work or a time at home when normally you would have a snack.

Changing eating habits is always a challenge, and especially so if you do not have the support of family and friends. Therefore, it is important to enlist the assistance of as many as you can. Explain to family, friends, and coworkers what you are trying to accomplish and why it is important. Give them specific suggestions for how they can help you. For example, ask family members to cooperate with you when planning meals and snacks at home and shopping for groceries. If you find it easier to exercise regularly when you have a partner, ask a friend to join you. When your friends or coworkers are deciding which restaurant to go to, request that they choose one that has options that are on your diet.

As you design your weight-reduction program, set reasonable goals. Remember, the objective is not to have a quick, dramatic loss of weight but to reach a healthy weight you can sustain for the rest of your life. This means that you should aim for modest losses every week or so. Set reasonable goals for implementing the changes in your routine. You do not have to tackle every problem area at once. Pick one aspect of your overall plan (e.g., eating more slowly) and focus on implementing it successfully before moving on to the next one.

As part of your program, establish a system of rewards for achieving your goals. Make a list of several items you would like to purchase for yourself and link each to one of your goals, or think of events or activities you would enjoy and make your participation in these events and activities contingent on achieving certain goals. You can even use dining at your favorite restaurant as a reward.

Finally, prepare for occasional setbacks. Even with the best of intentions and a well-designed weight-reduction program, you may not find it possible to always stick with your plan. When these lapses occur, do not make the mistake of giving up. View lapses as learning experiences, not as failures. Carefully review what happened and think of ways you can handle similar situations should they occur.

Suggestions for Congregational Programs
Sponsor a workshop on healthy eating and weight reduction led by a dietitian.
Organize a support group for individuals interested in losing weight.
Provide information about weight-reduction programs in the community.

Information Resources
https://www.niddk.nih.gov/health-information/health-communica tion-programs/win/Pages/default.aspx

A Brief Guide to Smoking Cessation

Smoking is the number one cause of preventable death in America.[2,3] Individuals who smoke have an increased risk of cancer, lung disease, heart attack, stroke, vascular disease, and even blindness, and have, on average, a life expectancy that is at least ten years shorter than that for nonsmokers. In spite of the well-documented link between smoking and these serious medical conditions, many people find it extremely difficult to quit smoking. The primary reason underlying this difficulty is that nicotine can be as addictive as cocaine or heroin.

Although stopping smoking can be difficult, the health benefits for those who succeed are significant and well worth the effort. For example, after one year your risk of coronary heart disease drops by 50 percent.

Knowing how difficult it is to overcome nicotine-related smoking addiction, individuals who decide to quit first need to develop a plan that takes into account the obstacles they are likely to encounter and the resources available to help them overcome these obstacles. This process starts by assessing your readiness.

- What is your motivation for stopping?
- What is likely to happen to you health-wise if you do not stop?
- What are the benefits if you can?

When listing benefits, start with the positive impact this will have on your health (e.g., living longer, reducing your risk of a heart attack, stroke, cancer, and lung disease), but be sure to include the benefits it will have on others (e.g., reducing their risk of diseases associated with secondhand smoke) and the financial benefits for you and your family as you spend less on tobacco products. Keep this list in a place where you can review it regularly.

Think through your daily routine and identify the various challenges you will face and the resources that are available.

- In what situations will the temptation to smoke be the greatest?
- What events are likely to trigger the urge to smoke?
- Has smoking been one of the ways you typically respond to stress or feelings of depression?

If you have tried to stop smoking before, review how you approached the challenge then and what interfered with your attempt(s), and understand that your chance of stopping forever increases with every attempt you make.

- What can you do differently this time?
- Who are the people most likely to discourage or interfere with your effort to quit smoking?
- Who are the individuals you will definitely be able to count on to support your effort?

As you begin to develop your smoking cessation plan, consult with your health care provider and inquire about medications that have been approved to help people stop smoking. Studies have shown that taking these medications can improve your chance of success. Make sure you understand how to use the medication and what side effects there might be. You also can ask if your provider knows of any hospital-sponsored smoking cessation programs or behavioral health professionals (e.g., psychologists or other mental health professionals) who specialize in working with individuals who are trying to stop smoking. If there are no programs or professionals in your community, telephone counseling is available at 1-800-QUIT-NOW.

The next step is to share your decision to quit and your motivation for quitting with family and friends. Request their support, offering them specific suggestions when you can. For example, ask those who smoke not to do so around you and those who do not smoke, especially the ones who did at one time but were able to quit, to provide encouragement for your efforts.

Because people often use smoking as a method of coping with stress, you may want to practice some stress management techniques before you stop smoking. Also build time and opportunities for more physical activity into your smoking cessation plan. This can help reduce stress and can also burn some of the extra calories if you find yourself eating more when you stop smoking.

Making changes in your home and work environment can help. Discard or move out of sight ashtrays and other items associated with smoking. Plan on changing your daily routine as well, and be sure to include pleasurable activities, especially ones that can help distract you when you have the urge to smoke.

Once you have identified the various challenges you will face, devised strategies for meeting these challenges, and pulled together the social resources (e.g., family, friends, and coworkers) and medical resources (e.g., medication) you will need, you are ready to stop smoking. The first few weeks are likely to be difficult, so during this time be sure to make good use of all the strategies and resources you have included in your plan (e.g., regularly review your list of reasons for stopping, spend time with your nonsmoking friends, and stay active). You also need to be prepared for setbacks—difficult or stressful situations where you are unable to resist the urge to smoke. If these occur, do not become discouraged and give up on your plan to quit smoking. Relapses are fairly common, even among highly motivated individuals, and do not mean that you will not be successful eventually. Use each setback as a learning experience and an opportunity to improve your plan. What situational or emotional cues seemed to trigger the smok-

The benefits of giving up smoking are so great that it is worth repeated efforts, and your likelihood of quitting for good goes up each time you try.

ing? How could you avoid these cues or handle them more effectively? Then start again. Remember, the benefits of giving up smoking are so great that it is worth repeated efforts, and your likelihood of quitting for good goes up each time you try.

Suggestions for Congregational Programs
Disseminate information about local smoking-cessation programs.
Sponsor a seminar on medications approved to help people stop smoking.

Information Resources
https://www.cdc.gov/tobacco/campaign/tips/quit-smoking/index
    .html?s_cid=OSH_tips_D9320
http://www.lung.org/stop-smoking/i-want-to-quit/

19

Managing Medications

Even individuals who have no signs of ill health can take many pre-scribed and over-the-counter medications to treat common conditions such as arthritis pain, high blood pressure, high cholesterol, and acid reflux. As people age and develop chronic diseases, the list of medications frequently grows long. But regardless of the number of medications a person takes, adverse side effects are always possible, and the risks increase dramatically as the number of medications rises.

While adverse reactions to medications occur frequently, noncompliance with prescribed medication regimens is probably even more common. Studies have shown that as many as 50 percent of patients fail to take their medi-cations as prescribed.[1] The problem is even greater for older adults, in large part because they are likely to have multiple chronic diseases and thus are prescribed many medications.[2]

Numerous factors contribute to the high incidence of noncompliance, and many can be traced to communication problems between

As many as 50 percent of patients fail to take their medications as pre-scribed.

patients and their health care providers. Often, patients do not understand why a certain medication has been prescribed. They may not understand its use and benefits and may be unaware of the risks of not taking the medica-tion as prescribed. Unpleasant side effects also can lead to noncompliance. Frequently, patients who experience unpleasant side effects stop taking the medication without informing their health care provider. Noncompliance also increases as the number of medications prescribed increases. Because elderly persons take an average of five to seven medications, it is not surprising that many have difficulty organizing and taking all of their medications as prescribed.[3] Finally, noncompliance can be related to economic status. Some medications are expensive, and individuals with limited financial resources may be forced to choose between buying a prescribed medicine and purchasing another needed product or service.

The Risks of Ignoring Information on Medication Management

The most serious danger of failing to take a medication as instructed is that the disorder or condition for which it is prescribed will not be well controlled, and thus an individual will be at risk of developing more serious medical problems. For example, people who have high blood pressure and fail to take their antihypertensive medications on a regular basis are increasing their chances of having a heart attack or a stroke. Another danger is that if people take some medications improperly, they may develop new medical problems, such as mental confusion or injuries sustained from a fall due to an imbalance related to adverse effects on brain function. Finally, even if one takes medications as prescribed, adverse drug reactions may still occur. Therefore, it is important for patients to understand the most frequent symptoms to watch for when starting a new medication and to always investigate with their health care provider or pharmacist whether new symptoms might be related to the medication they are taking.

Below is a brief guide to help people manage their prescription and nonprescription medications. This guide can be found on our website as well (www.hopkinsmedicine.org/jhbmc/building-hcp), and we recommend downloading and distributing it within your congregation.

Managing Medications

Medications can generally be managed effectively if you follow these recommendations:

- Understand why the medication has been prescribed. If you do not understand, you should ask. You should know what the medication is for, how to take it, and what to expect, including understanding common side effects or conditions that should prompt you to contact your health care provider.
- Take notes. Write down the information and instructions given by your provider. You should take notes about the prescribed medication while

you are in your provider's office. On our website are forms that can assist you in taking notes.

- Maintain a medication list. Keep an up-to-date list of all current prescription and nonprescription medications as well as any dietary or herbal supplements you are taking. This list should include the name of the medication, the dose you are taking, and how you are taking it. Also keep a record of any medication allergies. Bring this list to all medical appointments and to the pharmacy when having any new prescriptions filled. This list also should be available to family members or other caregivers. In the event of an emergency, this list can be referred to by health care providers. (A medication record sheet is available on our website.)

- Ask about foods and drinks that should be avoided while taking the medication(s).

- Ask your primary care provider to review all of your medications. Take your medications or your medication list to office visits, even to appointments with specialists. Remember, this includes over-the-counter (nonprescription) drugs, dietary supplements, and herbal remedies.

- Report any unexpected or unpleasant side effects to your health care provider.

- Use one pharmacist or pharmacy for all of your medications, and accept medication counseling when a pharmacist offers it. If you still have any questions about the medication, ask your pharmacist or the health care provider who prescribed the medication. In fact, by law, pharmacists are required to offer medication counseling whenever a prescription is dispensed.

- Ask your pharmacist to contact your provider or insurance company if you feel that you cannot afford the medication that has been prescribed. Oftentimes, there are alternatives covered by your insurance company that are just as effective as the original prescription. For example, in regard to asthma inhalers, there are more than a dozen steroid inhalers, and insurance companies may cover only one or two. If your health care provider prescribes one that the insurance company does not cover, ask for him or her to rewrite the prescription for the inhaler that the insurance company does cover. Your pharmacist can help with finding such alternatives.

- Take a trusted family member or friend with you if you have difficulty talking with your provider or pharmacist.
- Use medication organizers or pill boxes if you have trouble remembering to take your medicine. These inexpensive boxes can be purchased at pharmacies. Setting an alarm on your smart phone also is a good way to remind you to take your medication at the right time.
- Refill prescriptions in a timely manner so that you will not run out of your medications.

Suggestions for Congregational Programs

Sponsor a program or series of programs on medication management with a local pharmacist as a featured speaker. Among the topics that could be covered in a series on medications are communicating with your pharmacist and provider about medications, commonly prescribed drugs and common mistakes people make when taking these medications, and nonprescription medications.

Offer members of your congregation medication organizers. These organizers can be purchased at pharmacies or online. Some hospitals, home health agencies, and pharmacies may be willing to donate a small number of the organizers.

Distribute medication record forms and worksheets. Medication record forms and worksheets are available on our website (www.hopkinsmedicine .org/jhbmc/building-hcp) and can be downloaded and distributed to your congregation and at community programs. These materials can help people to better understand their medications and keep them organized.

Use congregational bulletins and mailings to remind members of your congregation of the need to take their medications as directed. Provide information on some commonly prescribed medications. This information can be obtained from our website or local hospitals and pharmacies. You also can include information on common adverse events and side effects.

Examples of Congregational Programs

At the Masjid Al Ihsan in Baltimore, an afternoon was spent teaching local congregation members about medications. The discussions were led by physicians and nurses, with ample time allowed for questions and answers. Among the topics covered were common side effects, dietary concerns, common food and drug interactions, and medication interactions. The difference between **generic medications** and **brand-name medications** (or trade name medications) as well as medication categories that include alternatives which can vary by insurance coverage were explained. Also, handouts that helped explain medication coverage and health insurance were provided. At the conclusion of the program, participants were given medication organizers that had been donated by several local pharmacies.

Asthma control is often dependent on using inhalers. However, using an inhaler can be more challenging than taking a pill. Therefore, during a back-to-school event sponsored by a diverse group of congregations, several physicians and pharmacy students were present to demonstrate to parents the proper use of an inhaler and what to do if their children encountered any problems. Several inhalers were brought in, and parents were invited to use them (as these inhalers were for demonstration purposes only and had no actual medication in them) in order to better understand exactly what is involved in their use. An important feature of this program was that because of the diversity within the group, the presentations were offered in English, Spanish, and Arabic.

Information Resources

The Food and Drug Administration has consumer education materials on its website: www.fda.gov/Drugs/ResourcesForYou/Consumers/default .htm.

Local pharmacies and hospitals can supply information sheets on various medications.

For more information and resources, along with additional examples of congregational health programs, please visit the book's website at www .hopkinsmedicine.org/jhbmc/building-hcp.

20

Preventing Accidents and Falls

Accidents and falls frequently are overlooked as major health problems associated with aging. However, both the number and severity of falls increase with age, and falls are the leading cause of fatal and nonfatal injuries for older adults. Each year almost 3 million older adults are treated in emergency departments for fall injuries, and more than 800,000 are hospitalized for these injuries.[1]

Many factors increase the risk of falls among older adults. Some of these are associated with the aging process, while others are associated with medical disorders (e.g., diabetes or stroke) that occur more frequently in old age. Such disorders can cause muscle weakness, sensory deficits, or balance problems that can lead to postural and gait instability. In addition, adverse reactions to many commonly prescribed medications can result in inattention, drowsiness, dizziness, or weakness and can directly cause a fall. Finally, many falls are the result of environmental factors that could be prevented if proper home inspections and modifications are made.

> **Each year almost 3 million older adults are treated in emergency departments for fall injuries, and more than 800,000 are hospitalized for these injuries.**

The Risks of Ignoring Information on Accidents and Falls

Besides the risk of severe head trauma and spinal cord injury that can be fatal, fall injuries can lead to fractures and brain injuries that often seriously limit a person's ability to carry out normal, everyday activities. Many people who have fallen and suffered injuries experience permanent problems with mobility, and one-year mortality rates among older persons following a hip fracture are likely 20–30 percent. In addition, the fear of falling that often follows a major injury may result in a reduction in activities, leading to muscle weakening and, paradoxically, possibly further increasing the risk of future falls.

What Can Be Done to Reduce the Risk of Accidents and Falls?

Fortunately, there are a number of changes that can be made in the living environments of older adults to reduce the risk of accidents and falls. These include:

- Removing throw rugs
- Tacking down large rugs and carpeting completely
- Using nonslip polish on floors
- Keeping objects off the floor
- Installing handrails along both sides of the stairs
- Providing good lighting on steps, landings, and any other particularly dark areas
- Placing light switches in easily accessible locations or using motion-sensor lighting
- Using nightlights in bedrooms, bathrooms, and hallways
- Using nonslip rubber mats in showers or baths
- Installing handrails for baths and toilets
- Keeping water off the floors
- Using adaptive equipment for baths or showers (e.g., seats or benches)
- Installing a raised toilet with side rails or using a bedside commode
- Keeping food and frequently used items where they can be reached without using a stool

People also can reduce the risk of accidents and falls by using assistive devices such as canes and walkers. It is important to encourage individuals who would benefit from such devices to use the most appropriate and effective ones, and to emphasize how they can help to prevent falls and serious, even life-threatening injuries. Health care providers can make a physical therapy referral to assess needs and assist with obtaining the appropriate assistive device.

Other steps you can take to lower your risk of falling include:

Exercise to improve your balance and strength. Lack of exercise leads to weakness and can increase your chance of falling. Practice exercises that improve balance and make your legs stronger to lower your risk.

Review your medications. As you get older, the way medications work in your body can change. Medicines or combinations of medicines can make you sleepy or dizzy and cause you to fall. It is important to report these symptoms to your health care provider. Ask your health provider or pharmacist to review the medicines you take—even the over-the-counter medicines. It might be helpful to bring all of your pill bottles with you to your next appointment. You also may want to ask if you would benefit from vitamin D.

Have your vision checked. Poor vision can increase your chance of falling. See an eye doctor at least once a year to have your vision checked and to update your eyeglass prescription. If you do get a new prescription, especially if you are switching from single-vision eyeglasses to bifocals or progressive lenses, take extra caution when walking or using steps the first few days, since it can take time to adjust to the changes in your vision. Looking through the bottom lens of bifocals may distort your perception. It is best to discuss with your optometrist if you should have separate glasses for distance and reading.

Suggestions for Congregational Programs

Sponsor a program on home safety, mobility, and assistive devices. A physical therapist could be one of your featured speakers, along with representatives from several companies that provide in-home medical supplies and equipment.

Check with your local health department or department on aging for programs they offer regarding falls, exercise, and balance.

Recruit and train a group of volunteers who would be willing to conduct home safety checks for members of the congregation. Social workers from a local hospital or a home health agency can assist in their training.

Recruit and train a group of volunteers who are willing to use their knowledge and skills to make minor home modifications based on home safety checks (e.g., install grab bars and handrails).

Recruit and train a group of volunteers who are willing to deliver meals to people with physical limitations. Another option is to connect these people with local agencies (e.g., Meals on Wheels) that can provide the service. This could help some individuals avoid or delay placement in a nursing home or other long-term care facility.

Organize a group of volunteers who are willing to provide basic house and yard maintenance for people who are physically incapacitated. This could be done on a short- or long-term basis, depending on the congregation's needs and resources. Seasonal activities such as lawn mowing, leaf raking, snow shoveling, or spring gardening help might be organized.

Use congregational bulletins and mailings to provide members with helpful suggestions and reminders about home safety. Educational materials can be obtained from the national organizations included in the Information Resources section of this chapter. Also, home health agencies and companies that provide in-home medical supplies and equipment may have materials that you can distribute.

Example of a Congregational Program

An excellent example of a program designed to reduce accidents and falls is one that was sponsored by Florida Hospital DeLand and several local congregations. Invitations to attend this free program, titled "Fall Prevention and Safety in the Home," were mailed to all religious congregations in DeLand and the surrounding community, and an announcement was placed in the religion section of the local newspaper. The program, held at a downtown church, attracted an audience of 60 and featured two physical therapists (one from the hospital's rehabilitation department and the other from the hospital's home health agency), a pharmacist, and a representative of a medical equipment company, all of whom were enthusiastic about participating.

The program began with the physical therapist from the home health agency reviewing various safety hazards frequently found in the home and offering suggestions for removing or avoiding these hazards. She was followed by the physical therapist from the rehabilitation department, who demonstrated exercises individuals could do in their homes to gain strength and improve their balance. The representative of the medical equipment company then demonstrated a number of assistive devices and types of mobility equipment, including canes, walkers, rollators (rolling walkers), transfer benches, scooters, and power chairs. The final presentation was by the pharmacist who reviewed the various types of medications that could increase the risk of falling. The presenters then fielded questions from the audience and also remained after the conclusion of the program to meet with several individuals who had additional questions.

Information Resources

Information and materials on preventing falls and accidents can be found on the website for the Centers for Disease Control and Prevention (www.cdc.gov/homeandrecreationalsafety/index.html).

The National Institute on Aging (NIA) also has materials on preventing falls that can be ordered or downloaded from the NIA website (www.nia.nih .gov/health/publication/falls-and-fractures).

For more information and resources, along with additional examples of congregational health programs, please visit the book's website at www .hopkinsmedicine.org/jhhmc/building-hcp.

21

Supporting Family
Caregivers

Families are being called on to play an increasingly important role in health care today. A recent survey conducted for the National Alliance for Caregiving and the AARP Public Policy Institute found that almost one of every five adults in the United States is serving as a family caregiver, a term that is used most often to describe individuals who care for members of their family of origin but also can refer to those who care for their family of choice—often a member of their congregation, neighbor, or close friend.[1] These informal, unpaid caregivers tend to the needs or concerns of persons with limitations caused by illness, injury, or disability.

Families are being called on to play an increasingly important role in health care today.

Almost any illness, injury, or medical condition can result in a person needing a family caregiver. Some individuals may require only temporary, short-term assistance while recovering from an injury or surgery, while others may need long-term care for a chronic disease. Health conditions that often lead to the need for a caregiver include:

- Alzheimer's disease and other dementias
- Cancer
- Chronic obstructive pulmonary disease (COPD)
- Heart failure
- Diabetes
- HIV/AIDS
- Injuries resulting from falls
- Kidney disease

- Multiple sclerosis (MS)
- Parkinson's disease
- Psychiatric disorders
- Severe arthritis
- Stroke
- Traumatic brain or spinal cord injury

Exactly what are family caregivers called on to do? Most help with at least one **Activity of Daily Living (ADL)**. These activities include getting in and out of beds and chairs, getting dressed, getting to and from the toilet, bathing or showering, feeding, or dealing with incontinence or diapers. And family caregivers help, on average, with more than four **Instrumental Activities of Daily Living (IADL)**. These include transportation, grocery or other shopping, housework, preparing meals, managing finances, giving medications, pills or injections, or arranging outside services. But family caregivers do more than assist with ADLs and IADLs. Increasingly, they are called on to monitor the health of their loved one, communicate with health care professionals, and advocate with providers and agencies. Many are performing tasks that are typically thought of as nursing tasks. These can include preparing and administering intravenous feedings, providing wound or ostomy care, using meters and monitors (e.g., glucometers, blood pressure monitors, oxygen saturation monitors), using incontinence equipment and supplies, and operating medical equipment (e.g., lifts, home dialysis equipment, suctioning equipment).

Most caregivers report that they have had little preparation for many of the tasks they take on, and providing this care can be physically and emotionally demanding, especially for those caring for loved ones with chronic mental health issues or Alzheimer's disease and other forms of dementia. It often means sacrificing some of their own interests and not paying enough attention to their own health. There is also often the challenge of balancing caregiving with work. It is not unusual for family caregivers to have to reduce their work hours or take a leave of absence, which then impacts their own financial situation.

Although it may seem obvious that family caregivers play a central role in health care today, their contributions are sometimes overlooked by health care systems, medical professionals, coworkers, and even some family members and friends. They often do not receive the recognition and gratitude they deserve or the preparation and support they need. Religious congregations interested in addressing these shortcomings will find it helpful to draw on the programs and materials developed by Johns Hopkins Bayview Medical Center's Called to Care program, a family caregiver initiative developed with the assistance and generous support of the Harry and Jeanette Weinberg Foundation. Especially helpful is the booklet developed for the program, *Called to Care: A Guide for Family and Friends*. Much of the remaining information in this chapter is taken from this booklet. A PDF of the entire booklet can be found on our website (www.hopkinsmedicine.org /jhbmc/building-hcp).

Helpful Tips for Caring for Your Loved One

Create a safe environment at home. One out of every three older adults falls each year. Almost 3 million are treated in emergency departments for fall-related injuries, and approximately 800,000 of these are hospitalized.[2] Given the high risk of falls, it is a good idea to conduct a safety inspection of your loved one's home. In fact, everyone should do this, especially if you have older adults who live with or visit you. More information about reducing the risk of accidents and falls in the home can be found in chapter 20.

Maintain medical records. Most care recipients take at least one prescription drug. It's important to keep a list of all medications (including over-the-counter drugs), as well as the dosage or strength, what condition the drug is treating, and how often it is taken. A drug regimen may change often, so be sure to make regular updates to this list.

Educate yourself. Learn about each disease or condition that your loved one has, its treatments, and the likely course of the disease. The more information you have, the more you will know what to expect and the better prepared you will be. The Johns Hopkins Health Library is a valuable resource that provides information on the diagnosis, treatment, and prevention of conditions. To access the library, visit www.hopkinsmedicine.org/healthli brary. You also may want to visit one of the websites included in chapter 25 for additional information on various diseases and treatments.

Communicate with health care providers. In order to be a good advocate for your loved one, you should understand the terminology used by health care providers. Do not be afraid to ask questions if you do not understand something that you hear or read. If you feel like the health care team doesn't fully understand your loved one's needs and concerns, speak up. It's critical that there is good two-way communication between patients and providers. You can play a valuable role helping with this.

Keep extended family involved and informed. Host a family meeting with all decision makers. Identify and discuss the issues of providing care for the family member in need. Come up with a plan to share responsibilities and to keep everyone updated regularly.

Ask for help. Caregiving can be time consuming and emotionally draining. Don't be afraid to ask for help! Finding ways to free yourself from some responsibilities can be helpful to both you and your care recipient. Remember to be specific when asking for assistance. For example, instead of saying, "I need some help with Dad," ask, "Can you stay with Dad for two hours on Friday so I can go to an important appointment?"

Manage your time. Keep an appointment book or calendar to schedule your daily activities, including visits to the doctor. Consider using an online calendar that can be shared with other family members.

Learn to be an effective caregiver. There are many resources available to help you become an effective caregiver. While some of your responsibilities may be common sense, others may require further education and training. For example, you may want to learn the safest way to transfer a loved one from a bed to a wheelchair. This can help prevent serious injury to yourself and your care recipient.

Transitions in Care: Navigating the Health Care Maze

Caregivers of individuals with a chronic illness experience increased stress during episodes of acute illness, which may require a transition from one care setting to another. Often, important health care decisions need to be made in a short period of time. There are a few guiding principles that apply to these likely occurrences. The following information can help guide you through that process.

Know your loved one's health insurance policy. Take time to understand the insurance coverage. You don't want any last-minute surprises. For example, many older Americans are not aware that Medicare does not cover the full cost of a hospital stay and other necessary care. Find out if your loved one qualifies for medical assistance and, if not, look into options for secondary insurance. Understand prescription coverage and copays for medication. Some insurance companies have case management programs to help navigate patients through chronic illness. Contact your loved one's insurance company to determine if this option is available.

Write it down. Use a caregiving journal to keep a detailed record of all aspects of your loved one's care.

- Include the names of all health care providers.
- Keep a list of current medications and side effects.
- When speaking with hospital staff and community agencies, write down names, phone numbers, dates, and what was said. Make sure that you are receiving information from the treatment team in the language with which you are most comfortable.

Talk about the tough stuff. By the time someone needs a caregiver, onset of a life-threatening illness is likely. It is important to talk about care plans and medical decisions well in advance. It's especially helpful to discuss advance directives and a financial power of attorney so that if a crisis happens, the care recipient's wishes are clear and you are able to uphold them. More information on advance directives can be found in chapter 16.

Develop and maintain a good relationship with your loved one's primary care provider. He or she can be instrumental in partnering with the hospital team if an admission is needed.

Start your involvement from day one of any hospitalization. If you are the caregiver of someone who has been admitted to the hospital, start getting involved in your loved one's care from the time of admission. Introduce yourself to the health care team, and share your loved one's care plan that was in place prior to being hospitalized. Be clear about any aspects of care that you are worried about or those where additional help may be needed.

Know your health care team. If the hospital is an academic medical center, such as Johns Hopkins Bayview or the Johns Hopkins Hospital, your loved one will be cared for by a team of health professionals. Members of this team often include an attending physician, fellow, resident physician, nurse practitioner or physician assistant, and medical student. Your loved one also may be cared for by a nurse, certified nursing assistant, and—if necessary—physical, occupational, or speech therapists.

It can be quite difficult and confusing to keep track of everyone who is caring for your loved one. We encourage you to speak up and let your team know if you are unclear about what the plan of care is or are uncertain about who will be involved providing that care.

Once your loved one is ready to transition from the hospital, a team of professionals will help coordinate additional care. The team, composed of a social worker, nurse case manager, and case assistant, is trained to help families through the difficult care decisions that arise at discharge from a hospital and to help them plan accordingly when there is a change in a patient's functional abilities. They will refer you to community resources, such as nursing homes and rehabilitation centers, home care services, medical equipment providers, and transportation services. The team also may be able to help with financial and legal concerns. It may be helpful to meet with this team early in the admission to start planning together.

Be firm, but flexible. Be firm. Speak up if you feel that a plan is not meeting your needs. You have the right to say no to a hospital discharge plan if you feel it is premature or if you are not prepared to manage the necessary care at home. If someone tells you that a particular service is not covered or available, take the time to see if the decision can be negotiated or formally appealed to an insurer. For patients covered by Medicare, information about appeals is provided on the Medicare website (www.medicare.gov).

Be flexible. You may not always find the perfect solution to a problem. Be willing to consider an alternate plan or a choice other than your preferred one. Recognize that often some services will require out-of-pocket payments. If you are unable to afford necessary care for your loved one, ask your treatment team to link you with a hospital financial counselor.

Caregiver Health: Taking Care of Yourself

One of the challenges we face as we work with those who have been called to care is convincing them to take good care of themselves. This is easy to understand. You may feel that you do not have a right to tend to your own needs when your loved one is seriously ill or experiencing physical limitations. And then there are the other responsibilities that can place demands on your time—a spouse, children, and work. But, to be an effective caregiver, you also need to take good care of yourself. If you neglect your own health, you run the risk of becoming ill and then not being able to care for your loved one. Here are some suggestions that we hope you will take to heart.

Take breaks from caregiving. Time away from caregiving responsibilities—often referred to as "respite"—is essential to your health, which can impact the health of your loved one. Although it may seem difficult to arrange these periods of respite, there are several options that might be available to you.

In-home respite care—Ask a family member or friend to stay with your loved one so you can take care of your own responsibilities or get together with friends. Some community organizations, including religious congregations, have volunteers who are trained to provide in-home respite care for a few hours. For a fee, home health services can provide a personal care aide to stay with your loved one.

Adult day centers—These centers provide daily care in a group setting for individuals who need supervision. If you need a longer period of respite, check with local nursing homes or assisted living facilities to see if they are able to care for your loved one for several days.

Leisurely activities—Use your "down time" to care for yourself. Do things that you enjoy and that reenergize you. Read a book, listen to music, or talk on the phone with a good friend.

Safeguard your own health and well-being.

- Go to your health care provider for regular checkups. Let your provider know that caregiving is an important part of your life. Make sure you mention any symptoms or concerns.
- Take your medications as prescribed and monitor your own health with the same attention you give your loved one.
- Get a flu shot. Supplies of the flu vaccine sometimes run short, so be sure to obtain one early in the flu season. You also may want to ask your provider if you should receive the pneumonia vaccine. Being vaccinated may keep you from getting sick as well as from infecting your loved one.
- Find time to exercise regularly. You don't need to join a gym or participate in exercise classes. Even short walks in your neighborhood can be beneficial to your physical and mental health.
- Take classes that focus on stress-reduction and coping techniques. You may find yoga, meditation, and other relaxation techniques particularly helpful.
- Engage in resilience-building activities. One example is taking a few minutes at the end of each day to list two or three things that went well and that you can feel good about accomplishing.
- Continue to participate in religious or spiritual activities, as well as recreational activities, sports, or hobbies. You may not be able to be as involved as you were previously, but it is important that you continue

to engage in at least some of the activities that meet your spiritual, emotional, and social needs.

Know your employee rights. If the demands of caregiving reach the point where they conflict with your work responsibilities, you may want to take advantage of the Family and Medical Leave Act (FMLA). This act allows eligible employees who work for an organization with 50 or more employees and who are caring for a spouse, parent, or child with a serious health condition to take up to 12 weeks of unpaid, job-protected leave from work. Government agencies and elementary and secondary schools also are covered by FMLA, regardless of the number of employees. To learn more about FMLA, visit the Department of Labor's website: www.dol.gov/whd/fmla/employeeguide.pdf.

Join a support group. It is not unusual to feel isolated when you are devoting so much of your time to caring for a loved one. One valuable way to overcome these feelings is to join a support group where you will find others who understand the stresses and challenges you are facing. Members also may offer valuable advice, coping strategies, and resources. Some support groups are designed for all caregivers, while others are for individuals who care for people with a particular medical condition.

NOTE: The demands of caregiving can be overwhelming, often putting the caregiver's own health at risk. It is not unusual for caregivers to experience stress-related disorders, including depression. If you are feeling down, depressed, or hopeless; have little interest in things you previously enjoyed; have trouble falling or staying asleep; have lost your appetite or have trouble concentrating, talk with your health care provider or a mental health professional. There are effective strategies and treatments that can help restore your energy and lift your spirits. More information on depression and its treatments can be found in chapter 12.

Suggestions for Congregational Programs

Find opportunities to recognize the contributions of family caregivers. The month of November, designated annually as National Family Caregivers Month, is an excellent time to express appreciation for family caregivers.

Remember to include family caregivers, as well as their loved ones, in the concerns and prayers of the congregation.

Provide assistance for family caregivers in need of respite care. One of the most frequently identified caregiver needs is for respite care, even if it is just to have someone stay with their loved one for two or three hours. Congregations can help by maintaining a list of respite care programs in the community. Also, some congregations may be able to offer their own program by partnering with a local hospital or social service organization to train and support volunteers who can offer brief, in-home respite care.

Provide assistance for family caregivers in need of emotional support. Congregations can assist by maintaining a list of support groups offered in the community. Some of these may be designed for all caregivers, while others may be for individuals who care for people with a specific medical condition (e.g., Alzheimer's disease).

Encourage family caregivers to take care of themselves. Many caregivers find it difficult to attend to their own physical, emotional, and spiritual needs, feeling guilty taking time for themselves when their loved ones are experiencing so many limitations. Encouragement from clergy and lay leaders can help relieve the guilt they might be feeling.

Examples of Congregational Programs

An outstanding example of a congregation offering support and resources for family caregivers is the Alvin and Lois Lapidus Center for Spirituality and Healing at the Beth El Congregation in Baltimore. This center, also known as the "Soul Center," was envisioned and founded by Rabbi Dana Saroken as a place people could come for workshops, seminars, support groups, or simply to meet and connect with others who are facing some of life's physical, emotional, or spiritual challenges. One such program is the monthly Caregiver Café that is offered in partnership with Jewish Community Services and Johns Hopkins Bayview Medical Center. From the moment caregivers enter the center, they see that they are genuinely appreciated and valued. They are greeted warmly by Rabbi Saroken, Rachel Siegal, director of the Soul Center, and Linda Stewart, director of Johns Hopkins Bayview's Called to Care program, who offer to take their coats and to serve them a cup of coffee or tea. This is a time and place for them—the caregivers—to be on the receiving end of care and compassion. Once the group has gathered, Rabbi Saroken, Rachel, and Linda excuse themselves to allow for a smaller, more intimate group, but they will return when the discussion has ended to once again show their appreciation for caregivers by serving them snacks and providing newcomers with a gift bag. A clinical social worker from Jewish Community Services facilitates the group discussion, with Dr. Panagis

Galiatsatos, a Johns Hopkins Bayview physician (and coauthor), present as a resource. This is a time that they can talk openly and in confidence about their challenges and their feelings, and when they do, they often discover that others understand what they are going through. They realize that they are not alone on their caregiving journey, and often the more experienced caregivers can offer valuable advice and suggestions. They have the powerful experience of being understood, supported, and loved.

In addition to the café, the Soul Center offers several other programs of value to caregivers, including a monthly healing service led by Rabbi Saroken, where "anyone in need of healing or praying for your loved ones is welcome." Also offered several times each month are "Jewish Meditation Sits," gatherings that "allow you to step out of the busyness of your life and experience the benefits of being present in the moment and free of self-judgment."

Another example of a congregation offering support for family caregivers is a program at Kingdom Life Church in Baltimore led by Ms. Tonoah Hampton. A key part of this program is providing respite care. To help prepare for this, Ms. Hampton's husband, Lamonte, attended a 10-hour respite care training program offered as part of Johns Hopkins Bayview's Called to Care initiative. This training program, led by Linda Stewart and Candyce Norris, provided participants with the knowledge, skills, and resources needed to provide and/or coordinate in-home companion care. Shortly after completing this course, a need for respite care arose when two sisters in the congregation found themselves in a difficult situation. They felt it was important to attend the funeral service of a close friend, but they didn't want to leave their ailing father alone for the four hours they would be away. Ms. Hampton was able to arrange for in-home companion care that allowed the sisters to attend the funeral without feeling guilty or worrying about the safety of their father.

The Hamptons also discovered that much of what Lamonte had learned in the respite care training would prove to be quite helpful when Tonoah's grandfather, diagnosed with a terminal illness and experiencing memory problems, moved in with them for the last four months of his life. Remembering what he had learned in the program, Lamonte took several steps to make their home safer for him, and then they both used some of the activities he had learned to help keep Tonoah's grandfather physically and mentally engaged. For example, they kept pictures of him and his family nearby and would, from time to time, ask him to identify the individuals in the photos and tell stories about them. They found that what they had learned from the respite training course, combined with the support they received from the hospice program, enabled them to provide her grandfather with many meaningful experiences and a rich quality of life until his passing.

Information Resources

AARP Caregiver Resource Center—www.aarp.org/home-family/caregiv
ing/planning-and-resources
Caregiver Action Network—www.caregiveraction.org
Family Caregiver Alliance—www.caregiver.org
National Alliance for Caregiving—www.caregiving.org
Share the Care—www.sharethecare.org

For more information and resources, along with additional examples of congregational health programs, please visit the book's website at www .hopkinsmedicine.org/jhbmc/building-hcp.

III   INNOVATIONS IN TRAINING

22

Medical-Religious Partnerships

A Hospital Chaplain's Perspective

Paula Teague has been a valued partner in our work in Baltimore over the last six years. As the Senior Director of Spiritual Care and Chaplaincy for the Johns Hopkins Hospital and Johns Hopkins Bayview Medical Center, we have worked with her to strengthen our outreach not only to clergy who frequently visit their congregants in our hospitals but also to clergy in the community with whom we have not had close ties in the past. This has allowed Johns Hopkins to expand its partnerships in a variety of ways, particularly with churches with large African American and Hispanic/Latino congregations. The collaboration between our spiritual care team and our Healthy Community Partnership programs has been enriching for all. We asked Reverend Teague to reflect on her career as a hospital chaplain, describe the programs on clinical pastoral education she leads, and share her thoughts as a health system leader on how medical-religious partnerships can improve the health of a hospital's neighbors and neighborhoods.

The role of a hospital chaplain has changed considerably since 1979, when I began my training. Much of that change is the result of shorter hospital stays. In 1979, the average length of stay in a hospital was more than ten days. Today, the average length of stay at Johns Hopkins Bayview Medical Center, where I serve as Director of Spiritual Care and Chaplaincy, is approximately three days. Increasingly, patients are receiving their medical care in outpatient settings rather than hospitals, and more and more responsibility for managing medical conditions is falling on the shoulders of patients and their families. These and other changes in health care have created new challenges for Clinical Pastoral Education (CPE), a program that offers training not only for clergy interested in pursuing a career in chaplaincy but also for congregational clergy who want to strengthen their spiritual care skills.

Community Partners Clinical Pastoral Education, a program developed at Johns Hopkins Bayview, offers a way to respond to these changes in health care and to provide continuity of spiritual care across the continuum of health-related experiences, including wellness activities, disease prevention, illness management, acute care, and end-of-life care. The desired outcome is both a congregational leader who can join a congregant on his or her health journey as well as a professionally credentialed chaplain who understands and appreciates the role of the community in the life experience of the persons with whom they minister.

In this chapter, I offer an overview of the Community Partners CPE program and discuss the differences between traditional CPE and Community Partners CPE. I also give an outline of an effective curriculum for integrating spirituality and health on the continuum of spiritual care. Additionally, I introduce you to some of the students participating in the Community Partners CPE program and then end the chapter with narratives from a few of our Community Partners CPE trainees.

Clinical Pastoral Education

Clinical Pastoral Education is experiential education for the provision of respectful, culturally competent spiritual care. The essence of spiritual care is developing a relationship through which assessment of spiritual concerns can take place and interventions can be carried out. CPE is focused on assisting spiritual care providers in learning about themselves and how to build relationships that can lead to meaningful spiritual care interactions, learning how to assess persons using various behavioral science frameworks, and developing a toolkit of appropriate spiritual care interventions.

A standard CPE program has a minimum of 400 supervised hours. For 300 of these hours, a student provides direct spiritual care services. These hours are usually provided in one setting and focused on that setting alone. For example, a CPE unit in a medical center might have a student assigned to certain patient care areas and also require some on-call shifts. These service hours are determined by the scope of the institution. The remaining 100 hours in a CPE unit are designated as educational hours. Approximately 50 percent of these educational hours are held in the format of case presentations called verbatims. Twenty percent of the educational time is dedicated to sessions focused on theoretical material provided by experts or interdisciplinary team members, with another 20 percent devoted to unstructured time for group process and group dynamics learning. Finally, about 10 percent of the educational hours are individually focused learning sessions with the CPE supervisor.

The Community Partners CPE program is similar to the standard CPE program in that it maintains the accreditation requirement of a minimum of 400 hours in the same ratio of 300 service hours to 100 educational hours. The essence of CPE is also maintained in that there remains a focus on relationship building, assessment, and intervention. The features or nuances added to the Community Partners CPE program are:

Increased number of didactic information sessions. The educational hours for the Community Partners CPE unit are divided equally between expert-led instruction, case presentations, and unstructured group/individual supervision. The expert-led instructional sessions are expanded to include participation in a Lay Health Educator program sponsored by the Healthy Community Partnership. CPE students are instructed in three additional areas: **population health, trauma informed care**, and the professional role of clergy or faith leaders in health and wellness.

Verbatim presentations with a broad scope required for each case. During the program, each Community Partners CPE student gives three case presentations that integrate the instructional material that has been presented to the group. Regardless of the context in which an encounter occurs, it is expected that the Community Partners CPE trainee will view each person broadly, including that person's living situation, congregation or spiritual home, health care needs, and level of health engagement.

Redefined health system boundaries and responsibilities. The model of the past largely limits health care to the institutional perspective of care delivered in hospitals and outpatient clinics. The recent emphasis on population health takes health care well beyond hospital and clinic walls. The CPE students participate in providing spiritual care in this new context, working not only within the hospital, but also in physician offices, other outpatient settings, and with neighborhood/congregational partners.

Increased variety of patient, client, and community encounters.

- Johns Hopkins Home-based Medicine is a program for older adults with chronic medical conditions who have a difficult or impossible time physically coming to a physician's or other health professional's office. These patients receive skilled services, such as nursing, social work, and physical therapy in the home. Chaplain trainees accompany providers on home visits and also provide house calls independently.

- Hopkins ElderPlus, a Program of All-inclusive Care for the Elderly (PACE), is a voluntary health program designed to provide and coordinate all needed preventive, primary, acute, and long-term care services so that older individuals can continue living in their homes. Chaplain trainees are involved at ElderPlus for a morning each week, providing spiritual support individually and in group activities such as Bible studies and spirituality sessions.
- Creative Alternatives is an outpatient psychiatric program that serves adults who have serious and persistent mental illnesses and who have not benefited from traditional services. The program combines mental health treatment, rehabilitative services, and assistance with daily living. The chaplain intern, along with a staff member, leads a weekly spirituality group for patients.
- The Center for Addiction and Pregnancy (CAP) helps mothers and infants deal with the physical, emotional, and social problems caused by addiction. Chaplain interns offer group and individual counseling with the clients.
- The outpatient lung cancer clinic provides screenings and multidisciplinary meetings for patients. Chaplain interns participate in the weekly multidisciplinary clinic, where they provide information about chaplain services and offer individual sessions with participants.
- The Chemical Dependency Unit (CDU) is an inpatient medical unit that provides safe medical detoxification for those suffering with addiction. Chaplain interns offer group and individual interactions.
- The Aliki Initiative, named for its benefactor, Mrs. Aliki Perroti, allows young physicians to have a reduced caseload in order to develop a deeper understanding of each patient's living situation and social support system. Chaplain interns round with the Aliki service on an inpatient basis and make home visits.
- Chaplain interns participate in physician offices as cases are reviewed by the health care team. The team can make referrals to chaplains for home visits with patients who are struggling with chronic conditions. The goal

is increased patient ownership of their care. When appropriate, chaplain interns help patients connect to local congregations in order to enhance social and emotional support.

A community health event organized in partnership with a local congregation. The CPE student works with clergy to assess congregational needs and create a health event. The goal of these projects is to practice partnership in the community, develop a better understanding of each partner's contributions, and organize a health event that addresses the needs of the congregation.

Expanded assessment tools. The Community Partners CPE students are asked to look at their spiritual encounters from three additional assessment perspectives. The first is population health, including the population health pyramid, which illustrates the health care continuum from home to acute care. Social determinants of health are introduced as a framework for understanding congregational health. Other topics such as quality of life, equity in wellness, prevention of illness, and access to services are discussed. Ideas about health disparities and their impact on life span and treatment are introduced. Students are then asked to begin including these elements in their assessment of the spiritual well-being of persons.

Trauma informed care as part of the assessment means that the impact of adverse childhood events (ACEs) is determined for each person. Community Partners CPE students get their own ACE score before working with patients. This helps the trainee to begin to look at his or her own narrative about trauma as well as the narratives of those with whom they work. Community Partners CPE helps each trainee identify the particular trauma for a patient or congregant and how that trauma impacts health and wellness in his or her current situation.

The third additional assessment concept involves the spiritual care provider's assessment of the impact of clergy on the health of the congregation and community. There is little that has been written about the influence of the local congregational leader on health and wellness. Clergy and chaplains are more often associated with crisis and acute episodes. "Call the pastor" is uttered when there is urgency. The Community Partners CPE program does not deny that this is a key role of the professional spiritual care provider, but it adds to this role the potential influence of the congregational leader's words about health and well-being.

Expanded evaluation of spiritual care encounter tool. Community Partners CPE students use an evaluation tool called PARTNER to assess the impact of their spiritual care visits. The tool can be used in any setting and asks the provider of spiritual care to make sure that social context and health literacy and access, as well as engagement, are included in the overall measure of success of the visit. It is not enough to think about spiritual care within the confines of the visit itself. How will the interaction be a part of the person's overall spiritual journey?

P: Person with whom you visited—Was his or her social context taken into account in your visits? Did you focus on his or her spiritual and health journey broadly? Did you include the ACE score? How? What was the outcome?

A: Activities—Take each of your interventions—verbal and nonverbal—and discuss whether they were effective to support the patient's well-being. Would you do something differently?

R: Refer—Is there a community connection that should be made in this visit? Is there a clergyperson who should be included in the medical team's goal-of-care meetings?

T: Theological—Is there a theological metaphor, passage, or theme that seems to fit this interaction? How did you use this theme with the person in order to support his or her overall recovery or health journey?

N: (K)nowledge needed—What health information would be helpful to this person? Was there congregational support that could be provided to improve health literacy? Is there something a medical professional should know about a gap in medical information?

E: Engagement—What does this person need to do to be further engaged in his or her own health care? Is there a need for an advocate or health care agent? Is there a need for faith community support? Is there anything you can do to help facilitate more faith community interaction?

R: Review—What did you do well? What could you have improved in the visit? Name at least two aspects of your ministry that changed the overall sense of well-being for the person with whom you ministered?

Participant Profile

As of spring 2017, there have been six Community Partners CPE groups with a total of 27 participants. The groups have been diverse with respect to age, gender, race/ethnicity, and religion. Only three of the participants have become full-time chaplains. The rest have career goals of becoming congregational leaders or ordained clergy.

All of the trainees in all six Community Partners CPE groups said that the program met their expectations and learning needs. Students named outpatient assignments as important in developing their pastoral authority—the capacity to assert one's role and expertise in the care of persons—more than inpatient assignments. Students in later units asked for more time in the outpatient areas. The Lay Health Educator program was named as a major learning experience.

There were comments from exit interviews that seemed especially indicative of the learning that takes place. One student said, the program "has helped me to understand what occurred before they got to the hospital, and to know what they're going to face. It creates awareness."

"My congregation believes in 'divine' health. For a pastor to say that God takes care of health *and* each congregant has a responsibility to take care of health opened a new understanding."

"Through my experiences as a chaplain, I have seen firsthand that many of the reasons people end up in the hospital are preventable... [M]edical-religious partnerships offer an excellent vehicle for transmitting health information to community members, information that can help avert costly medical procedures, improve health, and save/extend lives."

Narratives about Community Health Events

Each participant in the program had responsibility for organizing a community health event. Following are several stories about these events.

Many students have organized a health fair. In the second Community Partners CPE cohort, two of the students worked together to hold a health fair at one student's United Methodist congregation. They had a variety of topics and various booths, which included information on heart disease, diabetes, and mental health, and there was an "ask a doc" option, where two physicians from Johns Hopkins Bayview were set up in a more private area. There also was a sleep study expert who could test for sleep apnea, plus a masseuse who offered brief chair massages. A food drive also was included in the event in order to share "plenty" with others. Activities for children were planned so that they could be attended to while their parents toured the booths. There were approximately 50 participants at the fair. One of the planners of the health fair shared that this event was a high point of her CPE experience. "It helped me to take initiative which I have used in so many ways since that time."

In the most recent Community Partners CPE class, one of the trainees who pastors a United Methodist church organized a session on depression led by a recognized expert on the topic. The program was held immediately after the Sunday worship service but was open to the community as well as the congregation. Approximately 40 individuals attended this health event. She reported that many in her congregation have been impacted by depression, and for the first time several felt permission to share their stories. She was quite pleased to hear this, since one of her major objectives in offering this program was to remove, or at least reduce, the stigma of a mental health diagnosis felt by so many, particularly those in churches. She knew that many religious individuals believe that if only they had more faith, depression or other mental health conditions would lift. One particular congregant shared with this CPE trainee that often she had not attended church services because of her depression. Though open about her treatment, she commented to her pastor that she still suffered with her condition. The CPE trainee shared that this was a first in her ministry there, learning the more authentic reason for an absence that, in turn, provided a way to connect more closely with her parishioner.

A student in the third cohort coordinated with his priest in a Catholic parish to offer several workshops on naming a health care agent—the person who would be authorized to make health care decisions should an individual be unable to do so because of an injury or illness. These "Who Will Speak for You?" workshops focused on providing basic information about why it was important to name a health care agent and who could serve in that capacity, responding to questions and concerns, and encouraging participants to complete the appropriate form. The goal was to provide information about naming a health care agent and to get as many members of the congregation as possible to name a health care agent. Though the number of participants was modest, 90 percent of them did, in fact, name a health care agent.

In the Community Partners CPE programs there has been the option to survey the congregation about their overall health and their interest in particular health topics. In the first cohort, a congregation identified cancer as their main topic. A prominent surgeon was recruited to meet with the group. He came on a Saturday morning to the sanctuary of an African American

Baptist church in the inner city of Baltimore and listened as one after another told their story of cancer. He was able to debunk myths about cancer, discuss symptoms, and offer advice on how to get treatment. Additionally, there was a nurse in the congregation who offered to work with the hospital's Healthy Community Partnership to provide additional support. It was a session that the church still remembers today.

In later cohorts of the Community Partners CPE program, a more formal assessment was developed. In the most recent group, a church congregation that meets in a local school was asked to complete the survey as background for an "ask a doc" session to be held later. This survey information was shared with the physician, who in turn took the top three topics and prepared some information while also being available for more general questions. The survey helped the doctor to prepare and directly address the congregation's most immediate concerns. It also primed the congregants to think about their questions for the physician.

The Community Partners CPE participants uniformly report that these health events open up conversations that otherwise would not have been held. They break down stereotypes and misconceptions about diseases, particularly mental health conditions. They improve the health literacy of congregations and have a meaningful, real-life impact by equipping and empowering participants to gain better control over their health, their illnesses, and their health care.

In conclusion, the Community Partners CPE program has broken new ground by providing a way for CPE students to learn about providing spiritual care as both a listener and an agent of social change and social justice. The Healthy Community Partnership, with its focus on the intersection of spirituality and health, provides a forum to address the social sins of health care disparities and to pursue health equity. Graduates of the program are better able to see the social context of a person's life that is impacting spirituality. They can navigate the health system as well as provide health information in the congregation and even the congregant's home. A clergyperson can join the health care journey at any juncture with a sense of familiarity and professional competence. And professional chaplains who graduate from the program go on to partner with the community and local clergy to provide better care inside the hospital as well as the neighborhoods surrounding it. These chaplains are prepared to engage medical teams by the bedside and as community educators and advocates.

23

Medical-Religious Partnerships

A Young Physician's Perspective

Panagis Galiatsatos, MD, a graduate of the University of Maryland School of Medicine, began a residency in Internal Medicine at Johns Hopkins Bayview Medical Center in 2010, a year before Daniel Hale, PhD, moved from DeLand, Florida, to Baltimore. One goal of Dr. Hale's relocation was to establish at a major teaching hospital the medical-religious partnership programs that he had developed as a faculty member at Stetson University in Florida and to explore how these programs could benefit physicians-in-training. The hope was that these programs would become a key part of the training curriculum, provide doctors with a richer understanding of their patients, and become a national model for improving medical education in the United States. Although Dr. Galiatsatos already had a strong interest in community outreach, he recognized that the medical-religious partnership programs offered a special opportunity to impact the lives of community residents and the physicians who provide their care, and he immediately assumed an active leadership role in these programs. We asked Dr. Galiatsatos to reflect on how his experiences with us have influenced his own training and development as a physician, as well as the careers of internal medicine residents who have followed him in the Johns Hopkins Bayview Medical Center internal medicine residency program.

For many of us in the medical profession, our commitment to a career in health care begins years before any official schooling or training. For me, it was evident as a youth that I desired to be a physician. This desire had its roots in the community where I was raised, which I imagine is true for many others. Growing up in Baltimore City, surrounded by family who emigrated from Greece as well as good friends who were long-time Baltimore City citizens, I felt a strong sense of community that enabled me to pursue this dream of becoming a physician. And my vision of the doctor I wanted to be encompassed, in one way or another, my ability to give back to the community. I knew I wanted to help create a social environment that promoted health, wellness, and a sense of meaning for all.

During college and medical school, as well as when we are interns and residents, many of us become less connected to our community. The detachment is not intentional; nor is it surprising, given the overwhelming amount of knowledge we must acquire and the long hours we must devote to our training. However, what is absolutely critical in defining our professional identity—namely, our patients—should remind us of the need for us to understand and engage with the community where they live and work. For me personally, engagement with the community not only was what I needed to do to become a skillful and effective physician; it also reignited the passion I once felt—the same passion that fueled my drive toward the health care field. And it started with a patient during my training as a resident physician.

Residency is a stage of graduate medical training when a resident, who holds a medical degree, practices medicine in a clinic and/or hospital under the direct supervision of a physician, called the attending. Residency is synonymous with long hours spent at the hospital and clinic, many medical procedures to master, and acquiring the ability to stay up to date with medicine's research breakthroughs. The training can be as short as three years and as long as ten or more years, depending on one's choice of specialty. This period in a physician's training is crucial. It is when our professional identity begins to take shape and typically culminated in a well-established identity that will be a part of us for years to come. Many factors influence the formation of a resident's identity but none more than the patients we encounter. And knowing a patient's community will further aid in shaping a physician-in-training's identity that will be suited to better serve patients in the twenty-first century.

Early in my residency it became obvious to me that mastering the pathophysiology of diseases was not going to fully result in the health and well-being my patients desired. The biological solutions I had to offer were often diminished or blocked entirely by the socioeconomic variables my patients faced every day in their homes and neighborhoods. For instance, in Baltimore City alone, neighborhoods with high poverty rates have high densities of

tobacco retail stores and, not surprisingly, higher rates of tobacco users. However, the assistance patients need to overcome socioeconomic barriers and
make significant progress toward achieving health equity goes well beyond
what can be provided by well-intentioned medical professionals operating
only within the confines of a hospital or clinic.

This is best exemplified by my patient, whom I credit with reinforcing my
belief in the need to train future physicians and other health care workers
to work with the community. Mr. H., a loving husband and father, and a
carpenter with many years of service, was admitted to my cardiac intensive
care unit with chest pain (he was suffering a massive myocardial infarction,
or a heart attack). His notes from the emergency department listed no prior
past medical history. I soon learned why—he had avoided going to the doctor and thus had never been properly screened for medical issues that likely
could have prevented his current medical condition. While he may have come
in with no medical diagnoses, he left with several: coronary artery disease,
heart failure, hypertension, hyperlipidemia, and type 2 diabetes mellitus.
This resulted in the need for him to take many medications (a total of 12
tablets daily). For me, it was clear that while he had become a great father,
husband, and productive member of the city's workforce, becoming a patient
would be his greatest challenge.

I paid him a home visit a few weeks after his discharge from the hospital.
We discussed a variety of things that afternoon, but my main concern was
how he was managing his new role as a patient. This is where I was most
shocked, the moment Mr. H. showed me his medication management: a jar
full of assorted pills and tablets. "I scoop out 12 medications a day, as I was
told," he said in a tone that lost its confidence once he saw my face. The great
values Mr. H. had acquired over his lifetime to serve his many roles did not
translate into becoming a patient. For example, his health literacy would be
one challenge for him in order to properly manage his diseases. The happy
ending to this story: to overcome his health literacy issues, we recruited his
family and his community (with the assistance of his pastor) to help him
manage his medications, as well as pick them up from the pharmacy, while he
recovered from his heart attack. The ability for a community to help its own
member resulted in my "eureka moment": medical-community partnerships.

This notion drove my colleagues and me ultimately to implement the
medical education initiative, Medicine for the Greater Good (MGG). MGG is
defined as a curriculum built on two pillars: first, educating resident physi-

cians about social disparities and their impact on health outcomes through lecture series and workshops. Second, much as physicians-in-training better understand a disease when they care for a patient who has that disease, physicians-in-training better understand the impact of health inequities by partnering with the community.

A challenge with community partnerships is with the definition of community itself. We realized early on in MGG that much of the data we have of the city was based on zip codes and neighborhoods. And while this is a good way to start to understand the health issues of a geographic region, it is limited in what it can contribute to a genuine understanding of the lives of those who reside within these regions. To gain this level of understanding, we would need to engage with a community with shared common characteristics and interests, and with an identifiable leader or representative who could assist with building a partnership with a hospital and its physicians. With an effective partnership established, health projects aligned with the community's health needs could begin to be developed. This structure could readily be established with the religious sector of Baltimore City.

Approaching communities, similar to approaching a patient, is not a "one-size-fits-all" solution. This is especially true when working with faith communities, in that most of the work occurs at their place of worship. Being mindful of customs, culture, and religious understandings is imperative in order to assure health goals are in accordance with spiritual beliefs and customs. As Congressman Elijah Cummings said at an MGG symposium in 2016, "You cannot lead where you do not go." Therefore, one of the strongest recommendations toward implementing a program that allows physicians-in-training to interact with the community is to visit congregations, let the members and leaders provide insight into the community, and even consider attending worship services.

There are two more advantages to having resident physicians work with the community. First, for physicians, as they go about their training from medical school to residency, it is well documented that the rate of "burnout" is high amongst them, compared to the general population. This feeling of burnout may even occur as early as medical school. From much of our work with the community through MGG, we have found through feedback and evaluations from residents and medical students that participation in community partnerships helps revive their calling to become physicians. Furthermore, it provides the residents insight into the health disparities within the communities they serve. While residents have limited ability to address major socioeconomic determinants of health such as poverty or homelessness during their training, they can be part of long-term strategic initiatives established by hospitals to improve the health of its neighbors and neighborhoods, as well as gain knowledge and skills regarding how physicians can play a role in these efforts. These experiences can not only benefit the trainees and their current patients but also future patients in the communities where they will one day practice. Our residents have recognized these benefits by working within the neighborhoods around our hospital, and my belief is that many have experienced new joy in their practice of medicine through this work.

The second advantage in working with faith-based organizations is the opportunity to learn more about the religious and ethnic cultures of patients served by a hospital. When caring for patients in clinical settings, it may be hard to grasp how patients' own culture can impact their ability to manage their health. However, when a resident-in-training is immersed in the community, and can witness firsthand what community means for a person of the Catholic faith or of the Sikh religion, it may impact the way the physician cares for his or her future patients. In one of our health initiatives, a resident wrote in her evaluation that the interaction with community "has impacted how I approach my patients, and how insight into their faith allows for conversation pieces that have helped build trust." Certainly, being able to better understand who the patient is, as provided through the knowledge gained by working in their community, further helps sustain the physician-patient relationship that is so important in the care of all patients.

Working with the community has always been the right thing to do in regard to promoting health and wellness. However, now more than ever, in an age where health inequities have resulted in life expectancy gaps of more than 20 years, depending on where you live in the United States, working with the community is also the smart thing to do. Promoting health within the confines of a hospital and clinic cannot be the only solution we offer our patients who live with chronic diseases, many of which are controlled as much by lifestyle changes as they are by pharmacological remedies. For further information on how to implement medical-religious partnership health projects within your community, utilizing resident physicians, visit our website (https://medicineforthegreatergood.com/) for suggestions on a curriculum and examples of community work.

IV **RESOURCES**

24

Community Resources

Many illnesses and injuries can create significant challenges for people who want to maintain their independence. If they do not have family or friends who can step in to assist them physically or handle some of the everyday tasks and responsibilities required to live in the community, they may find it necessary to move to another setting. Even if the person has a spouse or shares a home with another potential caregiver, the prospect of moving to a less independent setting may arise. For individuals who are faced with these situations but prefer to stay in their own homes as long as possible, the key may be finding professionals and agencies in the community that can provide help. Because arranging such services can be a daunting challenge for individuals who are already frail or disabled, members of a faith community can help in several ways.

The easiest step for a faith community is to create and regularly update a list of community resources, including a brief description of the services provided and contact information for local agencies. In addition, the congregation can sponsor seminars or health fairs at which agencies share information about their services. These programs give members of the congregation an opportunity to learn about community resources *before* they or family members need the services. Finally, members in some congregations, particularly those who have a background in health care or human services, may provide direct assistance to some congregants in need by taking on some of the everyday responsibilities (e.g., transportation, shopping, etc.), perhaps organizing groups or teams that can share these responsibilities.

Developing a list of community resources can be done very easily. A good way to begin is to contact the case management or social work department of your local hospital. The professionals in these departments are generally aware of the various services in the community. They should be able to provide you with a list of many of the services and programs, along with information about which services are likely to be covered by Medicare or other insurance policies, including the typical eligibility requirements for coverage.

Another excellent resource is your Area Agency on Aging. Established by the Older Americans Act of 1965, there are more than 600 Area Agencies on Aging. Some not only provide direct home- and community-based services to older adults but also support services for caregivers. To locate the Area Agency on Aging in your community, you can call 1-800-677-1116 or go to the Eldercare locator (www.eldercare.gov/Eldercare.NET/Public/Index.aspx), a public service of the US Administration on Aging.

Another good source of information about community agencies and programs is your local chapter of the United Way. Each chapter has a list of affiliates or partner agencies, many of which offer services for individuals with functional impairment. The location of your local United Way can be found by going to www.unitedway.org. Many United Way chapters are involved in establishing and supporting the 211 helpline. In communities with this program, people can call 211 to obtain information about health and human services. Services vary from community to community but often include food banks, rent assistance, Meals on Wheels, respite care, adult day care, and homemaker services.

An additional source of information about services in many communities is the local chapter of AARP. This organization also offers materials on a number of topics individuals and families with disease- or injury-related limitations are likely to encounter. Among the topics offered are caregiving, home modifications to improve safety, housing choices, legal issues, and driver safety. You can obtain these materials and information about your state and local chapters by visiting AARP's website: www.aarp.org.

The consumer beneficiary website offered by Medicare (www.medicare .gov) has information about health-related services in your community. This site allows you to list and compare the hospitals, skilled nursing facilities (nursing homes), home health agencies, health plans, and suppliers of medical equipment by state, county, or even zip code. Another source of information is your city or county social services department, which serves to promote individual well-being, protect vulnerable adults from abuse and neglect, and provide support to help people maintain their independence.

Transportation

One of the problems facing many individuals who have functional limitations and are living alone is transportation. They may be unable to drive themselves to medical appointments or to do basic shopping, and their health-related limitations may prevent them from using regular public transportation. In many communities the public transportation agency is able to provide door-to-door transportation for such individuals. Members of a congregational health ministry team can contact your local transportation agency to see if this service is offered in your community and, if so, how this transportation can be arranged. This information also may be available through your local Area Agency on Aging. Additionally, some home care or personal care agencies offer transportation services. Experienced case managers also suggest contacting a dialysis center or your local hospital's social work department and inquiring about the transportation services their clients use. Most state health departments offer transportation assistance to low-income residents through a Medicaid transportation program, which can include stretcher, wheelchair, or taxi access. You also may want to explore the ability of some of the more recent car transportation companies (e.g., Uber, Lyft) to assist individuals with special needs.

Assistive Devices

People with functional limitations are often able to continue living in their homes and maintain their independence if they have appropriate assistive devices. These can include grab bars in the bathroom, bath and shower chairs, handheld shower heads, raised toilet seats, transfer benches, bed grips, and lift chairs or cushions. Mobility aids, ranging from canes to motorized wheelchairs, also can help people maintain their functional independence. The congregational health ministry team can help individuals experiencing functional limitations by creating a list of local businesses that sell or rent this equipment. If local businesses do not carry all the items people need, there is the option of finding online businesses that have a comprehensive inventory of assistive devices. A related service that a congregation can offer is sponsoring a program at which an occupational therapist or other health professional familiar with assistive devices can demonstrate their proper usage. Many assistive devices are covered under health insurance. People can talk with their primary care provider to obtain a prescription for some assistive devices.

Home Modifications

It may be necessary in some cases for individuals to modify certain features of their home if they are to continue living there. A ramp may need to be installed if they are using a wheelchair or have difficulty climbing steps, and doorways may need to be widened to accommodate a walker or wheelchair. The installation of better lighting and handrails, along with the removal of throw rugs, can reduce the risk of falls. Congregational health ministry team members can help by identifying contractors who have experience making these types of modifications. A good place to find these contractors is a local medical supply business that carries assistive devices and other durable medical equipment. Many communities have home modification programs that can be accessed through the state agency responsible for disability services.

Personal Emergency Response Systems

A personal emergency response system, also called a medical alert system, can provide a sense of security for individuals living alone and their loved ones. These systems allow persons who are experiencing an emergency to summon help by simply pressing a button on a small radio transmitter carried in their pocket or worn around their neck or on their wrist. With some systems this sends a signal to a console connected to the user's telephone that automatically dials an emergency response center, where the operator determines the nature of the emergency and notifies the appropriate party from a list provided by the client (e.g., neighbor, family member, ambulance). Some emergency response centers are operated by hospitals, home care groups, or social service agencies; others are operated by the system manufacturer. Also available are systems where the console automatically calls the programmed phone number of a family member or friend, defaulting to 911 if the family member or friend cannot be reached. Members of a congregational health ministry team can help identify the options available in their community.

Meal Programs

Meals on Wheels, a program that provides nutritious meals for homebound individuals unable to prepare their own, operates in virtually every community in the United States. Information about local programs can be obtained from the website of Meals on Wheels America (www.mealsonwheel samerica.org) or from your Area Agency on Aging. Many communities also offer congregate dining programs for older adults who have a need for improved nutrition and socialization. Your Area Agency on Aging should be able to provide information about these congregate dining sites. People on fixed incomes also may be eligible for nutrition assistance through the local social services department.

Personal Care or Homemaker Services

In most communities there are organizations or businesses that provide nonmedical care for individuals who need assistance with some of their everyday responsibilities and activities. These services enable individuals to remain in their own homes and continue many of their routines and activities. Among the services offered by these organizations are meal preparation and cleanup, light housekeeping, laundry, changing linens, assisting with pet care, grocery shopping, incidental transportation, and escorting to appointments, meetings, and religious services. In addition to compiling a list of these organizations in your community, congregations can sponsor programs at which representatives of these organizations discuss the services they offer. Often local nursing schools can be a resource to link students who are available to help with nonskilled homemaker services.

Home Health Care

Individuals who need certain types of health care but are homebound or normally unable to leave home unassisted may require the services of a home health agency. Home health agencies provide and help coordinate the care ordered by a physician. These organizations offer a range of skilled care services, including physical and occupational therapy, speech-language therapy, wound care, intravenous or nutrition therapy, injections, and patient and caregiver education. Information about the home health agencies in your community and eligibility for Medicare coverage of these services is available at www.medicare.gov.

Support Groups

The challenges of living with the limitations and uncertainties of a chronic illness can leave the affected individuals, and sometimes their caregivers, feeling overwhelmed, emotionally drained, and deeply discouraged about their long-term prospects. Support groups, in which people facing similar health concerns and challenges gather on a regular basis, give individuals an opportunity to share their feelings and learn how to cope with the most difficult aspects of their situation. Members often receive assistance with the practical as well as emotional aspects of their illnesses, learning new problem-solving strategies and discovering additional community resources.

Identifying the various support groups in most communities can be challenging. Although some hospitals and community organizations maintain a list of support groups, in many communities there is no comprehensive list. A good place to start your research into this matter is to visit the website of your local hospital or contact the hospital's case management or social work department to see if they have a list of support groups. If they do not have a list, you will need to use your local library or the Internet to compile a list. You can start by visiting the websites of national organizations associated with specific conditions (e.g., Alzheimer's Association, American Cancer Society, Mental Health America). Many of these include contact information about support groups throughout the country or links to local chapters that have information about support groups. Another strategy is to call physicians' offices. For example, neurologists may be aware of support groups for those who have had a stroke or have Parkinson's disease, and oncologists may have information about cancer support groups. Additionally, many primary care clinics have begun to integrate the provision of behavioral health care into their medical practices to promote the overall physical and emotional well-being of the people for whom they care.

Financial Counseling and Assistance

For some individuals, handling basic finances can be a problem. Although they may have adequate resources, they find it difficult to handle certain financial responsibilities. In some communities the Area Agency on Aging or another community agency can arrange for a financial care manager or daily money management program to assume these responsibilities—making deposits, writing checks to pay the client's bills, and balancing checkbooks and bank statements. Clients can still maintain the responsibility for directing which bills should be paid and signing the checks. Another option is to arrange for a bank to electronically pay bills from the customer's account. The customer or a family member can monitor the account via the bank's online service—checking account activity and balances, viewing statements online, viewing images of paid checks, and transferring funds between accounts. The congregational health ministry team can explore various options and publish a list of organizations that provide these services.

Legal Services

Affected individuals or their families may need to obtain legal assistance for a number of illness-related challenges. These include Medicare claims and appeals, disability claims and appeals, guardianships, and disability planning, including the use of durable power of attorney, living wills, and other means of delegating management and decision making in the case of incapacity. As with many issues, the best time to learn about these is well in advance of a crisis. It is helpful for a congregational health ministry team to identify local attorneys who have experience in these areas of law and invite them to speak at a seminar.

Respite Care and Adult Day Care

For many individuals, their ability to remain in their own home depends largely on having a spouse or other family member live with them and provide much of their care. This arrangement often works well, but it can place considerable stress on caregivers who may find they do not have enough time to take care of their own responsibilities or that the strain of caregiving is jeopardizing their own physical or mental health. When this occurs, caregivers can consider several options to relieve some of the stress. For those who are capable of providing most of the care for a loved one but need some time away to tend to their own responsibilities and needs, respite care can be a good option. Some respite care programs provide an in-home companion, while others have a facility where the person in need of care can stay for a few hours. In some communities, organizations serving older adults have partnered with religious congregations to offer respite programs. When family caregivers need to go out of town for a few days or require medical treatment that will temporarily prevent them from providing care, skilled nursing facilities may be able to provide respite care. When individuals with a debilitating chronic illness cannot be left alone but the family caregiver has full-time work responsibilities, adult day care centers that offer a protective and supportive setting may be the best alternative.

The congregational health ministry team can provide a valuable service by exploring respite care and adult day care services in the community. Your research can start by contacting the Area Agency on Aging or the case management or social work department of your local hospital, but it also can include visiting programs to evaluate their facilities and services. Some congregations may want to explore offering their facilities and providing volunteers for a respite care program one or two days a week; if so, it is advisable to work closely with experienced professionals (e.g., hospital administrators, Area Agency on Aging staff) to ensure that the facilities meet any appropriate regulatory and licensing requirements, the environment is safe, and volunteers are properly trained. Another option is for a congregation to work with health and social services professionals to train volunteers to provide in-home companion care.

Care Management

For some individuals with chronic illnesses, the extent of their impairment and the services they require to live independently are not readily apparent. In such cases, the services of a care manager may be helpful. Geriatric care managers are health or human services professionals who can assess an individual's medical and human services needs and then assist in making arrangements for the provision of the required services. Care managers also can make regular visits to monitor the care and status of their clients, determining if any new challenges have arisen and additional services should be considered. Should the time come that the client is no longer able to live independently, the care manager can assist in finding the most appropriate living arrangement. The services of a care manager can be especially helpful when the family members who have assumed responsibility for the care of a loved one live in a distant community. To identify a geriatric care manager in your community, you can contact your local Area Agency on Aging or visit the website for the Aging Life Care Association (www.aginglifecare.org).

Palliative Care

Many seriously ill individuals are not aware of the benefits of palliative care or have the mistaken belief that it is only for those with a terminal illness. In fact, palliative care, with its goal of preventing or easing suffering and improving the quality of life for both patient and family, is appropriate for anyone experiencing pain and discomfort associated with their illness or its treatment. Palliative care typically is provided by a team of professionals—physicians, nurses, pharmacists, social workers, chaplains, and nutritionists—specially trained to treat distressing symptoms such as pain, fatigue, nausea, loss of appetite, sleep problems, and the emotional distress that can accompany a serious illness. Palliative care specialists are also experts in communication and skilled in helping patients and families navigate the uncertainties associated with serious illness. It is important for patients to understand that they do not have to give up their own health care provider and treatment plans or the goal of pursuing a cure for their illness in order to get palliative care. The palliative care team will work with, not replace, the patient's primary treatment provider.

Because so many people are not knowledgeable about palliative care, a congregational health ministry team can provide a valuable service by sponsoring a program on palliative care. This program would be especially helpful for clergy and congregational volunteers involved in visiting those who are seriously ill. Additional information about palliative care, along with a directory of palliative care providers, can be found at www.getpalliativecare.org.

Long-Term Care Resources

There may come a time when individuals find that they are no longer able to live independently or that their quality of life will be better if they move to a community or facility that can provide more comprehensive care and greater security. A congregational health ministry team can assist these individuals by compiling a list of the various options in the community that combine housing and services, as well as information about the types of services provided, costs, and approaches to financing. Four long-term care options are available in most communities.

Continuing Care Retirement Community (CCRC) or Life Care Community. These communities combine independent living, assisted living, and skilled nursing care in one setting. Individuals can start off living independently in their own apartment, townhouse, or cottage and then add services (e.g., meals, housekeeping, and transportation) or transfer to an on-site assisted living or skilled nursing care facility as their needs change. Many of these communities offer on-site primary and preventive health care services. Residents generally pay an entry fee and then monthly maintenance fees. Entry fees, policies on refunds of entry fees, monthly maintenance fees, and the fees for additional services and amenities vary widely. The cost of CCRCs are usually prohibitive except for the very affluent.

Assisted Living Facility (ALF). These facilities are generally appropriate for individuals who need assistance with activities of daily living but do not require skilled nursing care. The types of services and levels of care can vary, but they typically include assistance with meal preparation, household chores, managing medications, dressing, bathing, and even incontinence care. Some facilities arrange for transportation and offer regular social programs and activities. Almost 1 million people now live in ALFs, and costs range from $3,000 to $6,000 per month.

Skilled Nursing Facility or Long Term Care Facility (SNF or LTCF). These facilities, previously called nursing homes, are appropriate for individuals who require the services of registered nurses (RNs) and other licensed professionals on a daily basis. A majority of older adults will spend some time in a skilled nursing facility at some point in their life, oftentimes for a few days or weeks following a hospitalization while rehabilitating from an illness or injury. Others may spend many months or even years in this setting because of physical, cognitive, or emotional conditions that require complex medical, nursing, and personal care. Skilled nursing facilities provide a room (private or shared), all meals, 24-hour nursing supervision, access to needed medical services, personal care, and generally some social activities. A physician supervises the medical care of residents. Almost 1.3 million people reside in LTCFs, and at any given time 10–20 percent of residents are there for just a few weeks to recover and receive rehabilitation following hospitalization for an acute event or injury such as a stroke or hip fracture.

Hospice. Hospice care is appropriate when the goal of an individual with a terminal illness has shifted from cure or life-prolonging treatment to care aimed at relieving pain and controlling symptoms and supporting an individual and family through the dying process. Most hospices accept patients who have a life expectancy of six months or less if their disease runs its normal course (the requirement for Medicare reimbursement). Hospice care is provided by a team that includes physicians, nurses, social workers, chaplains, pharmacists, home health aides, and volunteers. Support is provided to the patient's loved ones as well. This care can be given in a person's home, in a nursing home, or in a residential care center.

Hospice services continue to be underused, with many eligible individuals never using hospice care and others electing it only in their final days or weeks of life. At least some of this underuse is the result of misunderstandings about hospice care. Some people believe it is only for individuals who have cancer or AIDS, and others assume it is appropriate only when death is imminent. In fact, hospice is often appropriate for individuals who have conditions such as COPD, heart failure, stroke, advanced liver disease, end-stage kidney disease, or dementia. Congregational health ministry teams can perform an important service by educating their congregations and communities about the nature of hospice care, the medical conditions for which it might be appropriate, and the point at which individuals and families may want to consider electing hospice care.

25

National Organizations

and Resources

There are numerous organizations that have excellent materials and other resources that can be used in planning congregational and community health programs. In this chapter we offer information about some of the ones we have found particularly helpful.

Health Ministries Association

The Health Ministries Association (HMA) is a nonprofit membership organization with a mission to "encourage, support and empower leaders in the integration of faith and health in local communities." The organization includes faith community nurses (formerly called parish nurses), health ministers, program leaders, and spiritual leaders. The HMA embraces people of diverse faiths, backgrounds, and interests and currently has approximately 500 members.

The HMA provides a number of benefits for its members, including an annual conference, representation to the American Nurses Association for the specialty practice of faith community nursing, discounts for HMA-developed resources, including *The Health Minister Role: Foundational and Curriculum Elements* and the *Faith Community Nursing: Scope and Standards of Practice*, consultation and support, a newsletter, a regularly updated website, toolkits and guides, discounts on HMA and other conferences, discounts on selected publications from partnering organizations, and opportunities for networking.

In addition to participating in the activities and events offered by the national organization, members can join and participate in activities and events offered by the constituency groups—faith community nursing, health ministry, program leadership, and spiritual leadership—and regional networks. The HMA website, open to both members and nonmembers, provides links to faith groups and other organizations that have programs and materials appropriate for congregational health ministries. For more information about the HMA, including how to become a member, you can visit its website (www.hmassoc.org) or call 1-800-723-4291.

Internet Resources

The Internet is the gateway to endless amounts of information. It's easy to use, accessible to most, and finds what you are looking for in a matter of seconds. With this in mind, it is no surprise that more and more people are tossing aside books and relying on the Internet as their main source of information.

There are thousands upon thousands of health-related websites. Keep in mind, however, that since the Internet is a public domain source, anyone can create a site regardless of their credibility. We suggest you follow these quick tips when searching the Internet for health information:

- Don't search the entire Internet. Start with Johns Hopkins Medicine Health Library or https://MedlinePlus.gov.
- Evaluate commercial ("dot com") sites carefully for bias and conflict of interest.
- Check to see if the information is current (less than three years old).
- Look for the credentials of the author (e.g., doctor, nurse, psychologist) to make sure the information is written by a health professional.

MedlinePlus (https://medlineplus.gov/)

MedlinePlus is a service of the National Institutes of Health and the US National Library of Medicine, the world's largest medical library. It offers information for patients and their family and friends on more than 1,000 diseases, illnesses, health conditions, and wellness issues. These topics are organized both alphabetically and by categories (e.g., Body Location / Systems, Disorders and Conditions, Diagnosis and Therapy, Demographic Groups, and Health and Wellness). For each topic, an overview or summary, the latest news, and links to the websites of other federal agencies and health-related organizations are provided. This website also has a medical dictionary, an illustrated medical encyclopedia, interactive tutorials, videos, and information on drugs and supplements. Information is provided in Spanish as well as English. MedlinePlus contains both copyrighted and noncopyrighted material. Noncopyrighted material (e.g., government information at National Library of Medicine websites) can be reproduced and redistributed without permission, but reproductions should contain proper acknowledgment of the source.

National Institutes of Health (www.nih.gov)

The National Institutes of Health's website offers information on hundreds of consumer health topics. For each topic, it provides links to websites that provide information and allow you to download information sheets, brochures, or booklets that may be reproduced and copied without permission. For example, selecting "Depression" will take you to the website for the National Institute of Mental Health, where you will find a 32-page booklet, *Depression: What You Need to Know*, which can be downloaded and copied. Selecting "Learn What a Heart Attack Feels Like—It Could Save Your Life" will link you to the website for the National Heart, Lung, and Blood Institute and a colorful two-page handout that illustrates what a heart attack feels like and what you should do if you believe you might be experiencing a heart attack. Many of the resources are available in Spanish as well as in English.

National Health Information Center (www.health.gov/nhic/)

The National Health Information Center (NHIC) is a health information referral service established by the Office of Disease Prevention and Health Promotion within the US Department of Health and Human Services. The NHIC website provides links to numerous governmental and private health-related organizations. Also available on the NHIC website is a comprehensive list of national health observances. Examples of observances are:

- American Heart Month
- Mental Health Month
- National Autism Awareness Month
- National Minority Health Month

Additionally, there is an extensive list of toll-free numbers for organizations that provide health-related information, education, and support. Examples of these organizations are:

- Alzheimer's Association Helpline
- American Childhood Cancer Association
- National Hispanic Family Health Helpline
- National Alliance on Mental Illness

Centers for Disease Control and Prevention (www.cdc.gov)

The Centers for Disease Control and Prevention (CDC), a part of the US Department of Health and Human Services, has as one of its major goals ensuring that people are healthy in every stage of life. As part of its strategy to meet this goal, the CDC provides on its website fact sheets and other informational materials on a number of preventive care measures that can be downloaded and copied. Many of these materials are available in Spanish as well as in English. Examples of topics are:

- ADHD Fact Sheet
- Preventing Falls: A Guide to Implementing Effective Community-Based Fall Prevention Programs
- Why Get a Flu Vaccine?
- You Can Control Your Asthma

HealthyChildren.org (www.healthychildren.org)

HealthyChildren.org is a parenting website sponsored by the American Academy of Pediatrics (AAP). The site, available in Spanish as well as English, offers health information organized by ages and stages—prenatal, baby, toddler, preschool, grade school, teen, young adult—and by health topic. Examples of health topics are:

- Allergies and Asthma
- Ear infections
- Eating disorders
- Immunizations

National Institute on Aging (www.nia.nih.gov)

The National Institute on Aging (NIA) produces a variety of informational materials on age-related topics for the general public. NIA's AGE PAGES are brief, easy-to-read information sheets on topics of interest to older adults and those who live or work with them. Examples of topics are:

- Dietary Supplements
- Forgetfulness: Knowing When to Ask for Help
- Heart Health
- Skin Care and Aging

NIA also produces lengthier publications on age-related topics. Examples of topics are:

- End of Life: Helping with Comfort and Care
- Long-Distance Caregiving: Twenty Questions and Answers
- Talking with Your Doctor: A Guide for Older People
- Understanding Alzheimer's Disease: What You Need to Know

Both types of publications may be downloaded and copied. Many of these materials are available in Spanish as well as in English.

Glossary

Activities of daily living (ADLs): Self-care activities that most people do without any assistance. There are six common ADLs including: eating, bathing, continence (controlling bladder and bowel functions), dressing, transferring (e.g., getting in and out of bed or chair without assistance), and toileting.

Advance directive: A written statement of an individual's desires regarding medical treatment, made to assure that his or her wishes are followed in a situation where the person has lost the capacity to make decisions or express his or her wishes.

Alveoli: Tiny air sacs of the lungs where air and blood can exchange particles (oxygen from air and carbon dioxide from the blood).

Alzheimer's disease: A chronic disease occurring later in life (middle or old age), brought on by a generalized degeneration of the brain. A type of dementia.

Angina pectoris: Chest pain or discomfort resulting from reduced blood flow to the heart muscle.

Asthma: A condition of the lungs where the airways (known as the bronchi) narrow (also known as spasms) and obstruct the ability of air to exit the lungs, resulting in the symptom of difficulty breathing. Airway spasms can be caused by exposure to allergens such as inhaled dust or ingested food, be triggered by acute infection, or occur with vigorous exercise.

Atherosclerosis: The hardening and narrowing of arteries (blood vessels that transport blood away from the heart), that in turn reduces the flow of blood to the body's organs. Symptoms develop (e.g., chest pain from a heart attack) when the flow of blood is stopped or severely reduced.

Attention deficit / hyperactivity disorder (ADHD): A behavior disorder marked by symptoms of difficulty maintaining attention, hyperactivity, and impulsivity.

Autism spectrum disorder (ASD): A group of disorders of development, often recognized in the first two years of life, that are associated with difficulty communicating and interacting with others, repetitive behaviors, and limited interests and activities.

Autoimmune disorder: Diseases where the cells of the immune system produce antibodies (proteins made by immune cells), or sometimes the immune system's own cells, attack the substances naturally present in the body. Examples of autoimmune disorders include lupus and rheumatoid arthritis.

Body mass index (BMI): A calculation that takes into account a person's height and weight, often used by health professionals to determine if an individual is overweight or obese. (See **Obesity**.)

Brand-name medication: Medications that have a trade name (e.g., Lyrica) and are protected by patents, resulting in the medications only being made and sold by the companies that possess the patents.

Cardiopulmonary resuscitation (CPR): A life-saving emergency procedure that includes external chest compressions, ensuring the heart continues to pump blood, and delivery of breaths, in an effort to aid the patient in breathing, provided when normal blood flow and breathing have stopped because of a catastrophic event such as a heart attack, electrocution, or drowning.

Caregiver: A person, paid or unpaid, who provides care for others with health and/or functional impairments.

Cataracts: A clouding of the lens of the eye that affects vision. Cataracts often develop slowly over time, with older age being a risk factor.

Chemotherapy: A category of drug therapies that use medications to destroy fast-growing cells (such as cancer cells). Chemotherapy includes medications swallowed in pill form or delivered in a liquid by injections or via a vein with intravenous fluids.

Chronic bronchitis: A condition of the lungs where there is inflammation and swelling of the lining of the bronchi (the airways of the lungs). The inflammation and swelling result in coughing, and often, excess mucus production.

Chronic kidney disease: A gradual loss in the function of the kidney over many years. It is identified using specific blood tests such as creatinine. Also referred to as **chronic renal failure**.

Chronic obstructive pulmonary disease (COPD): A condition of the lungs where airflow is chronically and significantly obstructed from leaving the lungs. This airflow limitation results in difficulty breathing and can be measured with pulmonary function tests. Emphysema and chronic bronchitis may cause COPD, but not all people with these conditions are diagnosed with COPD.

Colonoscopy: A test, often used for colorectal cancer screening, where a thin, flexible tube (a colonoscope) is inserted into the large intestine (colon and rectum) via the anus to evaluate the organ for any abnormalities (e.g., cancer, inflammation).

Compliance: Also known as adherence, refers to the degree to which a patient follows medical advice. May refer to medication (drug) compliance, device compliance (e.g., use of a walker), or lifestyle compliance (e.g., frequency of exercise).

Coronary artery disease: A disease of the heart where plaque builds up inside the heart's blood vessels, known as coronary arteries. The plaque buildup narrows the coronary arteries, limiting the amount of blood carrying oxygen and nutrients the heart muscle needs.

Delusion: A belief or impression that is maintained regardless of it being contradicted by evidence or a rational, logical argument.

Dementia: A clinical syndrome or condition in which there is a progressive deterioration of mental faculties, usually over many years. Memory problems are typically the first sign of dementia.

Depression (Major Depressive Disorder): A serious mood disorder in which a person has experienced five or more symptoms (defined in chapter 12) every day or almost every day during a two-week period, and at least one of the symptoms is depressed or irritable mood or loss of interest or pleasure in activities previously enjoyed.

Diabetes (type 1): A condition often presenting acutely where the pancreas has stopped making insulin (or is producing insulin in very low amounts). It is thought to be caused by an autoimmune process, and it is not linked to any modifiable risk factors (e.g., diet, obesity, physical inactivity). May be called by other names: insulin dependent diabetes or juvenile diabetes, as the condition often develops before adulthood.

Diabetes (type 2): A metabolic disorder, often with gradual onset, resulting from a variety of risk factors (e.g., genetics, diet, physical inactivity, obesity). Also known as adult-onset diabetes.

Diabetic ketoacidosis (DKA): A medical emergency and a complication of diabetes, whereby an individual's body produces high levels of ketones, resulting in the blood becoming acidotic, because of insufficient insulin in the blood.

Dialysis: A medical procedure using filters in an effort to function much like an "artificial kidney." Treatment removes fluid and waste products from the blood and ensures correct electrolyte (e.g., sodium, potassium) levels.

Diastolic blood pressure: The diastolic pressure is the bottom number in a blood pressure reading, corresponding to the minimal pressure in the arteries during the relaxation of the heart.

Elevated blood pressure: Blood pressure that is above normal but not at a level where it would be considered hypertension. The numbers include systolic pressure 120–129 mm Hg and diastolic pressure less than 80 mm Hg.

Emphysema: A condition of the lungs where the alveoli (air sacs of the lung) are damaged and enlarged. This may result in COPD if the lung damage is extensive.

Exacerbation: A sudden worsening of a chronic condition that can last for hours to days. Triggers to an exacerbation may be known (e.g., an infection) or unknown

Gastroesophageal reflux disease (GERD): Stomach acid and/or content flowing back into the esophagus. Over time, this backflow (or reflux) irritates the lining of the esophagus and can cause symptoms of chest pain or discomfort as well as the taste of acid or vomit in the mouth.

Generic medication: A medication equivalent to a brand-name medication with respect to dosage, route of administration, quality, performance, and intended use.

Glaucoma: A leading cause of blindness, glaucoma is a group of diseases that can damage the optic nerve. Often caused by abnormally high pressure in the eye.

Glucose: A simple sugar that functions as an important source of energy for the body and is always present in the blood.

Hallucination: A perception of an object or situation that does not, in fact, exist. Hallucinations can be auditory (heard), visual (seen), tactile (felt), gustatory (tasted), or olfactory (smelled).

Health care agent: A person chosen by an individual to make health care decisions when that individual has lost the ability to do so.

Health disparity: A health difference between populations that is closely related to disadvantages in economic, environmental, and/or social variables. Health disparities adversely impact certain populations who are defined by certain traits (e.g., race/ethnicity, religion, socioeconomic status, gender). Compare to **health equity**.

Health equity: This is the principle that highlights a commitment to reduce health disparities and the determinants of health disparities. Therefore, pursuing health equity means aiming for the highest possible standard of health for all persons, with more attention and resources allocated to those who are more disadvantaged. In other words, it means social justice in health and health outcomes. Compare to **health disparity**.

Health Insurance Portability and Accountability Act of 1996 (HIPAA): The Federal law that defined the rights of Americans related to health insurance and also included extensive requirements regarding Protected Health Information (PHI) and how it must be treated and secured.

Health literacy: The ability of a person to obtain, process, and understand health information and health services in order to make insightful and appropriate health decisions.

Heart failure: A condition whereby the heart cannot efficiently pump blood to the body.

Hemoglobin A1c (HgbA1c): A blood test that can be used to diagnose diabetes and prediabetes, as well as to monitor the effectiveness of diabetes treatment.

Hospice: A facility or service (often provided at home) where people with a terminal illness receive care, and support is given to their loved ones.

Human capital: A set of characteristics, such as knowledge and experience, as well as social and personality traits, that allows a person or group of people to engage in and perform acts that improve the condition of a community.

Hyperglycemia: An excess amount of glucose (sugar) in the blood at any given time. High blood sugar does not necessarily indicate that a person has diabetes, but if discovered the result requires further investigation to rule out a diagnosis of diabetes.

Hyperlipidemia: High levels of lipids (fats, cholesterol, and triglycerides) in the blood. A risk factor for developing atherosclerosis and coronary artery disease.

Hypertension: A chronic condition characterized by an increase in arterial blood pressure when measured using a blood pressure cuff, typically on the arm, and as defined by a systolic blood pressure (top number or first number) of 130 or greater and/or a diastolic blood pressure (bottom number or second number) of 80 or greater. Multiple blood pressure measurements are required to diagnose hypertension. Stage 1 hypertension is defined as systolic pressure of 130–139 mm Hg or diastolic pressure 80–89 mm Hg. Stage 2 hypertension is defined as systolic pressure of 140 mm Hg or greater or diastolic pressure 90 mm Hg or greater.

Hypothyroidism: A condition where a person's thyroid gland does not produce enough thyroid hormones (an underactive thyroid). The onset can be gradual over years, and symptoms are sometimes nonspecific, making diagnosis difficult. Unexplained tiredness and unusual swelling may prompt a test for hypothyroidism, and replacement hormone pills are available. (In contrast, hyperthyroidism, or an overproductive gland, can cause symptoms such as rapid heartbeats and extreme weight loss quite quickly.)

Incidence: The rate at which new cases of a medical condition affect a specified population over a specific period of time. For example, the annual rate of pregnancy for teenage girls in the United States was 56 per 1,000 in 2010. Compare **incidence** to **prevalence**.

Instrumental activities of daily living (IADLs): Skills that are needed to live independently and may be viewed as more complex than ADLs. These include handling transportation, managing money, shopping for groceries or other necessities, doing housework, preparing meals, managing medications, and using the telephone or other means of communication.

Insulin: The hormone made by the pancreas responsible for regulating the amount of glucose (sugar) in the blood.

Living will: A written document that details an individual's wishes and desires regarding medical treatment in circumstances where the individual can no longer make decisions or communicate his or her wishes regarding treatment. Compare **health care agent**.

Macular degeneration: Grouped as either wet or dry, it is a condition whereby the macula (a part of the retina of the eye) becomes injured, resulting in vision impairment (from blurry vision to blindness). In wet macular degeneration, blood vessels leak fluid into the macula. In dry macular degeneration, the macula becomes abnormally thin over time.

Mammogram: X-ray imaging of a woman's (or more rarely a man's) breasts to identify abnormal breast tissue and reduce the likelihood of breast cancer by detecting precancerous lesions (small areas of cells with microscopic abnormalities) when they can still be surgically removed for cure.

Melanoma: The most serious type of skin cancer, this is a type of cancer that develops from melanocytes (the cells of the body that contain melanin pigment, which give all people their characteristic skin color). Melanoma can develop in people of all ethnicities, though less darkly pigmented people of European descent are at highest risk.

Metabolic syndrome: A disorder including a group of risk factors that raise a person's likelihood for heart disease, stroke, and diabetes. The risk factors are: large waistline (greater than 40 inches for men, greater than 35 inches for women); a high triglyceride level; a low HDL (good) cholesterol level; high blood pressure; and high fasting blood glucose (sugar).

Metastasize: To develop cancer growth at locations away from the primary site of cancer. Cancer cells spread via the lymph (fluid circulatory) system and bloodstream. Common sites of metastatic tumors are in the liver, lung, bone, and brain.

Modifiable risk factors: Risk factors that can be changed and that affect an individual's risk of developing a disease. For example, weight, smoking status, alcohol consumption, and a sedentary lifestyle are modifiable risk factors.

Morbidity: The effects produced by a disease or illness that adversely impact function and well-being. For example, obese people can have symptoms of shortness of breath climbing stairs or aching joints because of the burden of excess weight from fat.

Myocardial infarction: Another term for "heart attack," where the blood flow to the heart muscle is blocked or severely limited and muscle damage results.

Nonmodifiable risk factors: Risk factors that cannot be changed and that affect an individual's risk of developing a disease. For example, a genetic condition, age, gender, and ethnicity.

Obesity (Overweight): A term to categorize individuals who have too much fat, often defined by the body mass index (BMI), a calculation that takes into account a person's height and weight. The Centers for Disease Control and Prevention defines a healthy BMI as 18.5–24.9; overweight as 25–29.9; and obese as 30 or more.

Palliative care: An approach, typically provided by a team of professionals, that has as its goal preventing or easing suffering and improving the quality of life for both patients and families.

Patient advocate: An individual, family member, or community member, paid or unpaid, who speaks on behalf of or aids in the health care of a patient or patients.

Peak-flow diary: A diary of the recordings of a patient's peak-flow meter. A peak-flow meter is a device that measures how well air moves out of one's lungs. If the numbers fluctuate from normal to low, such a finding may help a physician diagnose a patient with asthma.

Population health: A concept pertaining to improving community health that includes understanding the health and medical outcomes of a group of individuals, as well as focusing on strategies to improve the overall health of the specified population through not only medical care but also initiatives to address social determinants of health (e.g., education, job training, neighborhood safety).

Prediabetes: A condition characterized by a blood glucose (sugar) level higher than normal but not high enough to be diagnosed as having diabetes. Prediabetes is a risk factor for future development of type 2 diabetes and should serve as motivation to make meaningful lifestyle changes to prevent the progression to diabetes.

Prevalence: The percentage of a population who have or have had a specific medical condition at a specific point in time. For example, the prevalence of diabetes for all age groups worldwide was 2.5 percent in 2000. Compare **prevalence** to **incidence**.

Preventive medicine: A field of medicine dedicated to keeping people healthy and preventing, or at least greatly reducing, the risk of premature illness, disability, and death.

> **Primary prevention:** The goal of primary prevention is to prevent the development of a disease or disability.

> **Secondary prevention:** The goal of secondary prevention is to detect a disease as early as possible, thus allowing a greater potential for a cure or to slow its progression.

> **Tertiary prevention:** The goal of tertiary prevention is to reduce the complications and disabilities associated with an existing disease.

Pulmonary function tests: Tests intended to quantify how well the lungs exhale air and transfer oxygen from the air to the blood, as well as to measure the size of the lungs.

Rhinitis: An irritation or an inflammation of the mucus membranes of the nose. This may cause symptoms of a postnasal drip or rhinorrhea ("a runny nose").

Risk factors: Conditions that affect an individual's chances of developing a disease. These can be **modifiable** or **nonmodifiable**.

Screening: An approach intended to detect the potential presence of an unidentified disease, even if the patient is asymptomatic. Screening tests are often designed to identify a disease early, allowing for an intervention that ultimately reduces the morbidity (or adverse effects) from the disease, as well as the likelihood of death from the disease.

Social determinants of health: These are the conditions in the environments in which a person is born, grows, lives, works, and ages. The determinants are complex and include socioeconomic status and culture, education, physical environment, work status, social support system, and access to health care.

Stroke: A medical emergency, often called a "brain attack," it occurs when blood flow to part of the brain is interrupted or significantly reduced, and vital brain tissue is deprived of oxygen and vital nutrients, and subsequently, is irreversibly damaged. Common symptoms include difficulty speaking, and weakness or paralysis on one side of the body.

Systolic blood pressure: The systolic pressure is the top number or first number in a blood pressure reading, corresponding to the maximal pressure in the arteries during the moment the heart contracts.

Trauma informed care: An approach to caring for individuals who have experienced traumatic life events (e.g., violence, abuse, poverty, racism) where the treating health care professional is trained to understand the complexity of the impact of these events and thereby is better able to guide recovery.

Vaccination: Vaccines are preparations of a killed or modified microorganism, or more often, a constituent part of the microorganism, that can stimulate the body's immune response in order to prevent future infection. Vaccinations can prevent serious viral childhood diseases, as well as flu, pneumonia, and hepatitis in adults.

Vascular dementia: A type of dementia, also called multi-infarct dementia, that develops in older adults from the damage caused by poorly treated high blood pressure and atherosclerosis, whereby damage to brain tissue results from small strokes—some of which may not result in obvious symptoms when they occur.

References

Introduction

1. Centers for Disease Control and Prevention. *Chronic Diseases: The Leading Causes of Death and Disability in the United States.* 2017 [Accessed 21 August 2017]; available from: http://www.cdc.gov/chronicdisease/overview/index.htm.

2. National Center for Health Statistics. *Mortality in the United States, 2015.* 2016 [Accessed 21 August 2017]; available from: http://www.cdc.gov/nchs/data/databriefs /db267.pdf.

3. Colby, S. L., and J. M. Ortman. *Projection of the Size and Composition of the U.S. Population: 2014 to 2016. Current Population Reports, P25–1143, U.S. Census Bureau, Washington, D.C.* 2015 [Accessed 21 August 2017]; available from: http://www.census .gov/content/dam/Census/library/publications/2015/demo/p25-1143.pdf.

4. Centers for Disease Control and Prevention. *CDC Health Disparities and Inequalities Report—United States, 2013.* 2013 [Accessed 20 August 2017]; available from: http://www.cdc.gov/mmwr/pdf/other/su6203.pdf.

Chapter 4. Medical-Religious Partnerships and Community Health

1. Pew Forum on Religion and Public Life. *"Nones" on the Rise: One-in-Five Adults Have No Religious Affiliation.* 2012 [Accessed 21 August 2017]; available from: http:// www.pewforum.org/Unaffiliated/nones-on-the-rise.aspx.

2. Hartford Institute for Religion Research. *Fast Facts.* 2017 [Accessed 21 August 2017]; available from: http://hirr.hartsem.edu/research/fastfacts/fast_facts.html.

3. American Hospital Association. *AHA Hospital Statistics: 2017.* 2017 [Accessed 20 August 2017]; available from: http://www.aha.org/products-services/aha-hospi tal-statistics.shtml.

4. Putnam, R. *Bowling Alone: The Collapse and Revival of American Community.* 2000, New York: Simon & Schuster.

5. Putnam, R., and D. Campbell. *American Grace: How Religion Divides and Unites Us.* 2010, New York: Simon & Schuster.

6. Hale, W. D., and R. G. Bennett. *Addressing health needs of an aging society through medical-religious partnerships: what do clergy and laity think?* Gerontologist, 2003. **43**(6): pp. 925–30.

7. Baylor Institute for Studies of Religion. *The Baylor Religion Survey.* 2005, Waco, TX: Baylor University.

8. Centers for Disease Control and Prevention. *Disease Burden of Influenza.* 2017

[Accessed 21 August 2017]; available from: http://www.cdc.gov/flu/about/disease/burden.htm.

9. Centers for Disease Control and Prevention. *What You Should Know and Do this Flu Season If You Are 65 Years and Older.* 2017 [Accessed 21 August 2017]; available from: http://www.cdc.gov/flu/about/disease/65over.htm.

10. Lu, P. J., et al. *Racial and ethnic disparities in vaccination coverage among adult populations in the U.S.* Am J Prev Med, 2015. **49**(6 Suppl 4): pp. S412-25.

Chapter 5. Congregational Health Education Programs

1. Institute of Medicine. *Health Literacy: A Prescription to End Confusion.* 2004 [Accessed 21 August 2017]; available from: http://www.nationalacademies.org/hmd/~/media/Files/Report Files/2004/Health-Literacy-A-Prescription-to-End-Confusion/healthliteracyfinal.pdf.

2. Berkman, N. D., et al. *Low health literacy and health outcomes: an updated systematic review.* Ann Intern Med, 2011. **155**(2): pp. 97–107.

3. Boylan, A. M. *Sunday School: The Formation of an American Institution, 1790–1880.* 1988, New Haven: Yale University Press.

4. Anderson, J. D. *The Education of Blacks in the South, 1860–1935.* 1988, Chapel Hill: University of North Carolina Press.

5. DuBois, W. E. B. *Black Reconstruction: An Essay Toward a History of the Part Which Black Folk Played in the Attempt to Reconstruct Democracy in America, 1860–1880.* 1935, New York: Harcourt Brace and Company.

6. Ware, J., and J. Young. *Issues in the conceptualization and measurement of value placed on health,* in *Health: What Is It Worth?,* S. Mushkin and D. Dunlop, Editors. 1979, Pergamon Press: New York, pp. 141–66.

7. Rosenstock, I. M. *Historical origins of the health belief model.* Health Education Monographs, 1974. **2**: pp. 328–35.

8. Miller, W. R., and S. Rollnick. *Motivational Interviewing: Preparing People for Change.* 2nd ed. 2002, New York: Guilford Press.

9. Rollnick, S., W. R. Miller, and C. C. Butler. *Motivational Interviewing in Health Care: Helping Patients Change Behavior.* 2008, New York: Guilford Press.

Chapter 6. Coronary Artery Disease

1. Centers for Disease Control and Prevention. *Heart Disease.* 2017 [Accessed 3 August 2017]; available from: http://www.cdc.gov/heartdisease/.

2. National Heart Lung and Blood Institute. *What Is Coronary Heart Disease?* 2016 [Accessed 3 August 2017]; available from: http://www.nhlbi.nih.gov/health/health-topics/topics/cad.

Chapter 7. Hypertension

1. Whelton P.K., R.M. Carey, W.S. Aronow, et al. *ACC/AHA/AAPA/ABC/ACPM/AGS/ APhA/ASH/ASPC/NMA/PCNA Guideline for the Prevention, Detection, Evaluation, and Management of High Blood Pressure in Adults: A Report of the American College of Cardiology / American Heart Association Task Force on Clinical Practice Guidelines.* Hypertension. 2017, Nov 13. [Accessed 3 December 2017].

Chapter 8. Lung Disease

1. Centers for Disease Control and Prevention. *Asthma: Data, Statistics, and Surveillance.* 2016 [Accessed 3 September 2017]; available from: https://www.cdc.gov /asthma/asthmadata.htm.

2. Reddel, H. K., et al. *A summary of the new GINA strategy: a roadmap to asthma control.* Eur Respir J, 2015. **46**(3): pp. 622–39.

3. Vogelmeier, C. F., et al. *Global strategy for the diagnosis, management, and prevention of chronic obstructive lung disease 2017 report. GOLD executive summary.* Am J Respir Crit Care Med, 2017. **195**(5): pp. 557–82.

Chapter 9. Diabetes Mellitus

1. Centers for Disease Control and Prevention. *Diabetes: Data and Statistics.* 2017 [Accessed 21 August 2017]; available from: http://www.cdc.gov/diabetes/data/.

2. National Institute of Diabetes and Digestive and Kidney Diseases. *What Is Diabetes.* 2016 [Accessed 3 September 2017]; available from: https://www.niddk.nih.gov /health-information/diabetes.

3. Inzucchi, S. E. *Diagnosis of diabetes.* N Engl J Med, 2012. **367**(6): pp. 542–550.

Chapter 10. Kidney Disease

1. National Institute of Diabetes and Digestive and Kidney Diseases. *Chronic Kidney Disease.* 2017 [Accessed 22 August 2017]; available from: https://www.niddk.nih.gov /health-information/kidney-disease/chronic-kidney-disease-ckd.

2. Centers for Disease Control and Prevention. *National Chronic Kidney Disease Fact Sheet, 2017.* 2017 [Accessed 2 September 2017]; available from: https://www.cdc.gov /diabetes/pubs/pdf/kidney_factsheet.pdf.

Chapter 11. Cancer

1. National Cancer Institute. *Cancer Statistics.* 2017 [Accessed 21 August 2017]; available from: https://www.cancer.gov/about-cancer/understanding/statistics.

2. American Cancer Society. *American Cancer Society Guidelines for the Early Detection of Cancer.* 2017 [Accessed 22 August 2017]; available from: https://www.cancer .org/healthy/find-cancer-early/cancer-screening-guidelines/american-cancer-society-guidelines-for-the-early-detection-of-cancer.html.

Chapter 12. Depression

1. Centers for Disease Control and Prevention. *Current depression among adults—United States, 2006 and 2008.* MMWR Morb Mortal Wkly Rep, 2010. **59**(38): pp. 1229–35.

2. Kegler, S. R., D. M. Stone, and K. M. Holland. *Trends in suicide by level of urbanization—United States, 1999–2015.* MMWR Morb Mortal Wkly Rep, 2017. **66**(10): pp. 270–73.

Chapter 13. Dementia

1. Centers for Disease Control and Prevention. *Memory and Healthy Aging.* 2015 [Accessed 3 September 2017]; available from: https://www.cdc.gov/features/memory-healthy-aging/index.html.

2. Robinson, L., E. Tang, and J. P. Taylor. *Dementia: timely diagnosis and early intervention.* BMJ, 2015. **350**: p. h3029.

Chapter 14. Child and Adolescent Health Issues

1. Centers for Disease Control and Prevention. *CDC grand rounds: childhood obesity in the United States.* MMWR Morb Mortal Wkly Rep, 2011. **60**(2): pp. 42–46.

2. National Institute on Drug Abuse. *Principles of Adolescent Substance Use Disorder Treatment: A Research Based Guide.* 2014 [Accessed 27 August 2017]; available from: https://www.drugabuse.gov/publications/principles-adolescent-substance-use-disorder-treatment-research-based-guide/introduction.

3. Centers for Disease Control and Prevention. *Youth Risk Behavior Surveillance—United States, 2015.* 2015 [Accessed 27 August 2017]; available from: https://www.cdc.gov/healthyyouth/data/yrbs/pdf/2015/ss6506_updated.pdf.

Chapter 15. Vaccinations

1. Barberis, I., et al. *History and evolution of influenza control through vaccination: from the first monovalent vaccine to universal vaccines.* J Prev Med Hyg, 2016. **57**(3): pp. E115-E120.

2. Centers for Disease Control and Prevention. *Immunization Schedules.* 2017 [Accessed 28 August 2017]; available from: https://www.cdc.gov/vaccines/schedules/index.html.

Chapter 18. Modifying Common Risk Factors

1. Clarke, T. C., T. Norris, and J. S. Schiller. *Early Release of Selected Estimates Based on Data from 2016 National Health Interview Survey.* 2017 [Accessed 3 August 2017]; available from: https://www.cdc.gov/nchs/data/nhis/earlyrelease/earlyrelease201705.pdf.

2. Benjamin, R. M. *Exposure to tobacco smoke causes immediate damage: a report of the Surgeon General.* Public Health Rep, 2011. **126**(2): pp. 158–59.

3. Moritsugu, K. P. *The 2006 Report of the Surgeon General: the health consequences of involuntary exposure to tobacco smoke.* Am J Prev Med, 2007. **32**(6): pp. 542–43.

Chapter 19. Managing Medications

1. Lee, J. K., K. A. Grace, and A. J. Taylor. *Effect of a pharmacy care program on medication adherence and persistence, blood pressure, and low-density lipoprotein cholesterol: a randomized controlled trial.* JAMA, 2006. **296**(21): pp. 2563–71.

2. Brown, M. T., and J. K. Bussell. *Medication adherence: WHO cares?* Mayo Clin Proc, 2011. **86**(4): pp. 304–14.

3. Statista. *Prescriptions Per Capita in the U.S. in 2013, by Age Group.* 2017 [Accessed 3 September 2017]; available from: http://www.statista.com/statistics/315476/prescriptions-in-us-per-capita-by-age-group/.

Chapter 20. Preventing Accidents and Falls

1. Bergen, G., M. R. Stevens, and E. R. Burns. *Falls and fall injuries among adults aged >/= 65 years—United States, 2014.* MMWR Morb Mortal Wkly Rep, 2016. **65**(37): pp. 993–98.

Chapter 21. Supporting Family Caregivers

1. AARP Public Policy Institute. *2015 Report: Caregiving in the U.S.* 2015 [Accessed 3 September 2017]; available from: http://www.aarp.org/content/dam/aarp/ppi/2015/caregiving-in-the-united-states-2015-report-revised.pdf.

2. Bergen, G., M. R. Stevens, and E. R. Burns. *Falls and fall injuries among adults aged >/= 65 years—United States, 2014.* MMWR Morb Mortal Wkly Rep, 2016. **65**(37): pp. 993–98

Index

Baltimore City Health Department, 24, 27, 48

Baltimore Sun op-ed on depression, 114, 116–18

Barkin, Marshall, 147

barriers to care, 2, 4, 14, 57, 62, 208; depression, 112; language, 32; time or transportation, 49, 59; for vaccination, 138; for wellness promotion, 54–55

Baylor Religion Survey, 46

Bennett, Richard, 30

Beth El Congregation, 192

bipolar disorder, 108, 109–10

blood glucose level, 46, 95, 97, 231, 232, 234; diabetes and, 10–11, 12, 13, 69, 86, 87, 89–90; diet and, 92; exercise and, 89; hyperglycemia, 87, 232; insulin regulation of, 11, 90, 233; in prediabetes, 234; testing/monitoring of, 12, 13, 71, 88, 89, 90, 91

blood pressure, 75; categories of, 75; diastolic, 75, 231; elevated, 75, 231; screening, 20, 24, 27, 49–50, 62, 69, 76, 77–78, 97; systolic, 75, 235. *See also* hypertension

Body, Mind, and Soul health ministry, 9–22; background of, 14–16; curriculum of, 15; influence of, 21–22; skin cancer screening, 17–18, 49; topics covered by, 17–21; volunteer recruitment and training for, 15–16

body mass index (BMI), 69, 229, 234

Bowling Alone: The Collapse and Revival of American Community, 43

brain attack, 17, 235. *See also* stroke

brand-name vs. generic medications, 178, 230, 231

Breast Cancer Awareness Month, 57, 106

bronchitis, chronic, 80, 230

Brown, Christopher, 28

Buck, Tina, 16

Called to Care program, 30, 186, 192, 193

Campbell, David, 43, 44

cancer, 100–107; bladder, 104; Body, Mind, and Soul program for, 17–18; breast, 26, 49, 57, 68, 95, 100, 101–2, 104, 106, 107, 125, 233; cervical, 102, 104; colorectal, 49, 100, 102, 105, 230; congregational programs for, 105–7; deaths from, 1, 26, 100, 104; esophageal, 104; hospice care for, 18, 222; information resources on, 107; laryngeal, 104; lung, 100, 102, 104, 105, 106, 200; metastatic, 100, 234; obesity and, 100, 125; oral, 104; pancreatic, 104; prostate, 26, 95, 100, 103, 104, 106;

risks of ignoring information on, 101; screening for, 17–18, 26, 49, 100, 101–3, 106; self-examinations for, 17, 101, 103; skin, 17–18, 19–20, 46, 49, 100, 103, 106, 233; smoking and, 102, 104, 106; support groups for, 105, 106, 107; testicular, 103; treatment of, 105; warning signs of, 103–4

canes, 19, 180, 182, 215

cardiopulmonary resuscitation (CPR), 17, 45, 72, 74, 144, 230

Caregiver Action Network, 194

caregivers/caregiving, 1, 184–94, 230; Called to Care program for, 30, 186, 192, 193; congregational programs for, 191–94; for dementia, 18, 120, 121, 123; for depression, 113; health conditions requiring, 184–85; helpful tips for, 186–87; information resources for, 194; navigating transitions in care, 187–89; preparation and support for, 185–86; support groups for, 191, 192; taking care of oneself, 189–91, 192

care management, 220; financial, 218; geriatric, 220

Caring Connections, 148

car seats, 134

case management, 122, 187–88, 189, 213, 215, 218, 220

cataracts, 28, 89, 230

Center for Addiction and Pregnancy (CAP), 200

Center for Salud and Opportunities for Latinos (Centro SOL), 37, 40

Centers for Disease Control and Prevention (CDC), 48, 74, 79, 80, 93, 99, 107, 126, 129, 130, 131, 140–41, 183, 227

Chandler, Helen, 16

chaplains, 4, 5, 28, 197–205, 220, 222; Community Partners Clinical Pastoral Education program for, 198–205; PARTNER assessment tool for, 202

Chemical Dependency Unit (CDU), 200

chemotherapy, 16, 105, 137, 230

chest CT scan or X-ray, 81, 102

Chest Foundation, 85

chest pain, 17, 71, 72, 208, 229, 231

child and adolescent health, 125–35; asthma, 80–84; congregational programs for, 134–35; mental health, 127–31; obesity, 125–27; substance use disorders, 131–33; vaccinations, 136–41

Child Family Health International, 34

cholesterol level, 21, 232, 234; diet and, 70; heart disease and, 17, 20, 68; medications

ABOUT THE AUTHORS

W. Daniel Hale is a graduate of Florida State University and received his PhD in clinical psychology from the University of Massachusetts at Amherst, where he also completed his clinical internship. He served as a clinical psychologist at Orlando Regional Medical Center before joining the faculty of Stetson University, where he was professor of psychology and also director of the Community Health Initiative. In 1992 he began a collaboration with Dr. Bennett that has focused on the development of community-based health programs built around alliances between medical organizations and religious congregations. He joined Dr. Bennett at Johns Hopkins Bayview Medical Center in 2011, where he now serves as special advisor to the president. He also is an assistant professor of medicine in the division of geriatric medicine and gerontology and an assistant professor of psychiatry and behavioral sciences at the Johns Hopkins University School of Medicine. Dr. Hale is author (with Harold G. Koenig, MD) of *Healing Bodies and Souls: A Practical Guide for Congregations* and numerous research articles on mood disorders, aging, and chronic illness. He has served as president and executive director of the O'Neill Foundation for Community Health since 2003.

Richard G. Bennett is the president of Johns Hopkins Bayview Medical Center and a professor of medicine at the Johns Hopkins University School of Medicine. He is a graduate of Dartmouth College and the Johns Hopkins University School of Medicine. As a full-time faculty member at Johns Hopkins for more than 30 years, he was the Lublin Professor in Geriatric Medicine and served as executive medical director of the Johns Hopkins Geriatrics Center. He also served as the chief medical officer of Johns Hopkins Health Care from 1999 to 2003 and helped establish care management strategies embedded within multiple health insurance projects. In 2003, he was named vice president of medical affairs at Johns Hopkins Bayview Medical Center, and subsequently, executive vice president / chief operating officer, before being appointed president in 2009. Dr. Bennett is the author of dozens of professional journal articles and book chapters.

Panagis Galiatsatos is a graduate of Temple University and received his medical degree from the University of Maryland School of Medicine. His medical training was completed at Johns Hopkins Bayview Medical Center in internal medicine, followed by fellowships at the Johns Hopkins University in pulmonary medicine and the National Institutes of Health in critical care medicine. He joined the Johns Hopkins faculty in 2018. His research has focused on community health, health disparities, and resource allocation. In 2013, along with his colleagues, he established Medicine for the Greater Good at Johns Hopkins Bayview Medical Center and continues to serve as its codirector. Since 2011, he has worked with Dr. Hale in exploring the impact partnerships between religious institutions and medical organizations can have on the community and physicians-in-training, having published several research articles on these themes. Dr. Galiatsatos is the author of more than 30 research articles, and he has been the recipient of a number of awards, including the Martin Luther King Junior Community Service Award from the Johns Hopkins University and the Educational Program Award from the Institute for Excellence in Education at the Johns Hopkins University School of Medicine.